No More
Cellulite

No More
Cellulite

A Proven 8-week Program
for a Firmer, Fitter Body

**Wayne Westcott, Ph.D.,
and Rita La Rosa Loud**

A PERIGEE BOOK

A Perigee Book
Published by The Berkley Publishing Group
A division of Penguin Putnam Inc.
375 Hudson Street
New York, New York 10014

First edition: March 2003

Visit our website at www.penguinputnam.com

Library of Congress Cataloging-in-Publication Data

Westcott, Wayne L., 1949–
    No more cellulite : a proven 8 week program for a firmer, fitter body / Wayne Westcott, and Rita La Rosa Loud.— 1st Perigee ed.
      p.   cm.
    Includes index.
    ISBN 0-399-52857-1
    1. Cellulite.   2. Exercise for women.   3. Reducing diets.   4. Reducing exercises.
  I. Loud, Rita La Rosa.   II. Title.

RA778 .W258   2003
613.7'045—dc21

               2002035533

Printed in the United States of America

10 9 8 7 6 5 4 3 2 1

Dedication

WE gratefully dedicate this book to Jim Teatum, president of Nautilus, who prompted us to conduct our first program on cellulite reduction and has continued to encourage our research efforts in this important area of study.

Contents

Acknowledgments

WE are privileged to acknowledge the most valuable advice and assistance from Sheila Curry Oakes, our knowledgeable editor at Perigee. We greatly appreciate the excellent work of Marsha Young, our fitness administrative associate, in the preparation of this manuscript. Our special gratitude to Karen Leary for her professional expertise in designing the outstanding menu plan, and to William Humbert for his unmatched ability to package this information and so many other materials more artfully than we could ever imagine. We also thank our models, Olivia Chamberland, Tracy D'Arpino, Tricia Glynn, Marianne Kennedy, Susan Lovett, Maureen Minihan, and Taelese Piers for their expert demonstrations of the strength and stretching exercises. Our sincere appreciation to our supportive spouses, Claudia Westcott and Paul Loud, as well as to our gracious YMCA executives, Ralph Yohe, Mary Hurley, and William Johnson. We especially thank each of the participants in our numerous cellulite reduction research studies for their enthusiastic compliance with the exercise program, and our most helpful program instructors for doing such a great job educating and motivating their clients. We are most grateful to Barbara Harris and Linda Shelton, editors at *Shape* magazine, for their support and replication of our research studies. Finally, we humbly acknowledge God's grace in enabling us to initiate this work that we hope will help many women win their fight against cellulite.

Introduction

EVERY year, millions of women spend millions of dollars in an almost futile fight against cellulite. Even more amazing, scientists tell us that there is no such thing as cellulite. What women refer to as cellulite is simply fat, and it really shouldn't be a big deal. Yet any woman can tell you that cellulite isn't simply fat and that it *is* a big deal.

Why the discrepancy? If cellulite isn't just fat, then what is it? Perhaps more important, how do you get it? Certainly most critical, how do you get rid of it? While we definitely do not claim to have all the answers, we and our research staff at the South Shore YMCA have conducted enough studies on this topic to suggest a solution. Please note that the South Shore YMCA is a research facility where our highly trained staff conduct exercise/fitness studies with youth, adults, seniors, frail elderly, overweight individuals, advanced trainees, athletes, and disabled participants. Our research findings have led to the publication of almost 20 books and hundreds of articles on physical fitness, as well as book chapters/sections for the National Strength and Conditioning Association, the National Strength Professionals Association, the American Council on Exercise, the International Fitness Professionals Association, the YMCA of the USA, and the U.S. Navy.

We do not believe that the proper approach is another fat-reducing pill, powder, or formula. Nor do we think that you will receive any lasting benefit from creams, body wraps, rolling pins, or other devices that temporarily constrict or dehydrate the skin or reshape fat deposits. Our research-based recommendation for cellulite reduction is relatively simple, but it is not always easy to accomplish. It takes a little time, a little effort, and a little patience.

We have discovered that there are two major factors responsible for cellulite accumulation: muscle loss and fat gain. Our studies have confirmed that there are two essential requirements necessary for cellulite reduction: replacing the muscle tissue and reducing the fat stores. The purpose of this book is to give you general information for understanding and overcoming the cellulite problem, as well as to provide you with specific guidelines for attaining the desired results as safely, effectively, and efficiently as possible. We hope that the following chapters will help you to both decrease your cellulite deposits and increase your physical fitness so you look better, feel better, and function better as a result of a healthy and enhanced lifestyle.

If you follow our research-based exercise and nutrition program for 60 days, you might replace 1 to 2 pounds of firm muscle and lose 13 to 14 pounds of soft fat, for a major improvement in your cellulite condition and physical appearance. That is what some of our study participants achieved during their two-month training period. They did this with three 45-minute exercise sessions a week and by following a sensible/balanced nutrition plan. There is every reason to believe that you can do just as well, and perhaps achieve even better results.

1 | What Is Cellulite?

CELLULITE is the name given to the lumpy and bumpy, oatmeal appearance of legs and hips that have too much fat and too little muscle. It typically refers to the soft and saggy hips and thighs that plague so many women in our sedentary society. In order to understand what cellulite is and where it comes from, it is helpful to understand the structure and makeup of your legs and hips. The first and most obvious layer is our skin, which provides a protective covering for our body parts.

Just underneath the skin is our subcutaneous fat layer. Some areas of our body have relatively few fat cells, whereas other areas have lots of fat cells. For example, if you squeeze a fold of skin and fat on your forearm, it will most likely be pretty thin. This is because you have limited fat storage in this part of your body. However, if you squeeze a fold of skin and fat on your waist, hips, or thighs, it will undoubtedly be much thicker. This is due to the larger capacity for fat storage in these body areas.

Below the fat layer you will find your skeletal muscles. Ideally, your muscles should make up the majority of your limbs. For example, your thigh includes more than a dozen major muscles known collectively as the quadriceps (four muscles), hamstrings (four muscles), adductors (five muscles), and abductors (two muscles).

Your muscles surround and pull against the bones that comprise your skeletal system, such as the large femur bone in your thigh. Although bones are relatively dense and heavy, they represent much less mass than the muscles that control them.

Other notable tissues include tendons and fascia that attach muscles to bones, ligaments that connect bones to bones, blood vessels and blood that supply essential nutrients to all living tissues, and nerves that stimulate our muscles to contract and provide important feedback information to the brain.

Figure 1.1 offers a schematic diagram of the four major body components in the thigh of a well-conditioned young woman. You will see a thin skin layer, a slightly larger fat layer, and a massive muscle area surrounding a dense femur bone. This represents a firm, fit, trim, toned, and attractive thigh with no trace of cellulite.

Figure 1.2 offers a less-appealing schematic diagram of the same major body components in the thigh of an unfit middle-age woman. You will note a thin skin layer, a much larger fat layer, and a relatively small muscle area surrounding a less-dense femur bone. You will also notice that, unlike the smooth outer surface of the fit thigh, the skin appears irregular and wrinkled with the characteristic cottage-cheese appearance associated with cellulite.

We agree with the physiologists that there is no special tissue known as cellulite. It would seem that the soft and unattractively textured skin surface we refer to as cellulite is essentially the result of two factors, namely too little muscle and too much fat. Simply stated, when the underlying muscle layer becomes too thin

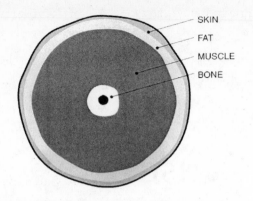

SKIN
FAT
MUSCLE
BONE

Figure 1.1

Cross-section of the four major components in the thigh of a well-conditioned young woman.

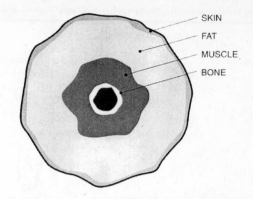

SKIN
FAT
MUSCLE
BONE

Figure 1.2

Cross-section of the four major components in the thigh of an unfit middle-age woman.

and the overlying fat layer becomes too thick, there is no firm foundation for the skin, which takes on the lumpy look of the formless fat layer beneath it. Unfortunately, these changes are the inevitable consequences of a sedentary lifestyle that have an insidious and undesirable impact on personal appearance and physical fitness.

2 | What Causes Cellulite?

As we age, our bodies undergo certain changes unless we take specific steps to delay the degenerative processes. Clearly, the most debilitating problem encountered during the mid-life years is the gradual loss of muscle. Most people are not even aware of the fact that they lose at least 5 pounds of muscle every decade of adult life. As illustrated in Figure 2.1, the average woman reduces her muscle mass by 5 pounds between the ages of 20 and 30, by 5 more pounds between the ages of 30 and 40, and by 5 additional pounds between the ages of 40 and 50. In fact, during the menopause years, the already alarming rate of muscle loss actually doubles. With such a rapid and cumulative reduction in muscle mass, it is not hard to understand why most 65-year-old women cannot lift a 10-pound weight.

Figure 2.1

Body weight and body composition changes during adult life.

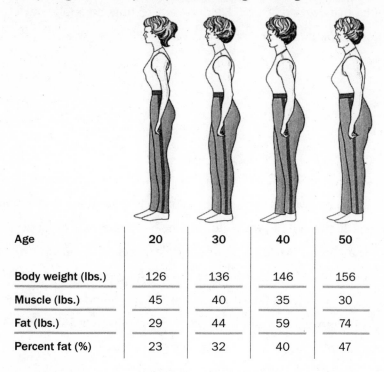

Age	20	30	40	50
Body weight (lbs.)	126	136	146	156
Muscle (lbs.)	45	40	35	30
Fat (lbs.)	29	44	59	74
Percent fat (%)	23	32	40	47

Muscle and Metabolism

Because muscle is very active tissue, it plays a major role in maintaining our metabolism. The more muscle you have, the higher your metabolic rate and the more calories you burn at rest as well as during physical activity. Conversely, the less muscle you have, the lower your metabolic rate and the fewer calories you burn at rest as well as during physical activity.

Generally speaking, the 5-pound-per-decade muscle loss results in a 5-percent-per-decade metabolic slowdown. The reduced metabolic rate means that the calories once used to keep the now atrophied muscle tissue alive and functional are no longer needed, so they are sent into fat storage areas.

You might not realize how large a role your resting metabolism plays in your daily energy utilization. Even if you are a physically active individual, most of the calories you burn every day are related to your resting metabolic rate. Muscle is a primary determinant of your resting metabolic rate, as illustrated in the following example.

Example

Tiffany and Tracy are both 20-year-old women who weigh exactly 100 pounds (see Table 2.1). However, Tiffany has more muscle than Tracy. As shown in Table 2.1, Tiffany is 20 percent fat, which means she has 20 pounds of fat weight and 80 pounds of lean weight. Assuming half of her lean weight is muscle (the other half consists of bone, blood, skin, connective tissue, and organs), she has 40 pounds of muscle. Tracy is 30 percent fat, which means she has 30 pounds of fat weight and 70 pounds of lean weight. Assuming half of her lean weight is muscle, she has 35 pounds of muscle.

Table 2.1

Comparison of body composition factors and resting metabolic rates for two young women with equal body weight.

	Body Weight	Percent Fat	Fat Weight	Muscle Weight	Resting Metabolism
Tracy	100 lbs	30 %	30 lbs	35 lbs	850 calories
Tiffany	100 lbs	20 %	20 lbs	40 lbs	1,075 calories
Difference	0 lbs	10 %	10 lbs	5 lbs	225 calories

Although a 5-pound difference in muscle mass might seem insignificant, note that Tiffany's resting metabolism is more than 200 calories per day higher than Tracy's resting metabolism. This represents a much greater energy requirement (6,000 more calories every month), making it much easier for Tiffany to maintain a desirable body weight while still eating plenty of food.

Actual Changes

Loss of muscle results in a lower metabolic rate, which leads to less energy utilization and more calories stored as fat. This decrease in muscle is really an insidious process that gradually puts on pounds without you knowing where they came from. After all, you're not eating as much food as you used to, and your lifestyle is about the same as it has been. How can you be losing muscle when your body weight keeps increasing?

As you saw in Figure 2.1 (p. 5), the average woman loses about 5 pounds of muscle every decade of her adult life. In addition, she adds about 15 pounds of fat every decade of her adult life. This results in a 10-pound weight gain every 10 years, disguising the facts that 5 pounds of muscle have been lost and that 15 pounds of fat have been gained.

Unfortunately, what the scale shows as a 10-pound weight gain is extremely misleading. Most people interpret this as a 10-pound problem, when in fact it represents a 20-pound problem. Rather than adding 10 pounds of fat, as indicated by the scale, you have actually gained 15 pounds of fat. Worse yet, the underlying cause of your fat gain is a 5-pound muscle loss. When you combine 15 pounds more fat and 5 pounds less muscle, you experience a 20-pound change in body composition, all in the wrong direction.

This is serious business, and it really takes a toll on a woman's health, fitness, and personal appearance by the time she reaches her forties and fifties. Take a closer look at Figure 2.1 (p. 5) We start with a well-proportioned 20-year-old woman who weighs 126 pounds. She has about 45 pounds of muscle and approximately 30 pounds of fat. This calculates to about 24 percent body fat, which is a desirable level for a healthy female of any age.

Now look at the same woman at 50 years of age. She has added 10 pounds of body weight each decade and now weighs 156 pounds instead of 126 pounds. She has 30 pounds of additional body weight, which she attributes to stored fat. If only this was true, we would undoubtedly have far fewer health concerns among middle-age women. However, she has actually added 45 pounds of fat and concurrently lost 15 pounds of muscle. This represents a 60-pound change in her body composition, which is almost half of her original body weight (126 pounds). Worse yet, she is now just under 50 percent body fat, which may predispose her to degenerative diseases and health problems such as high blood pressure, elevated cholesterol levels, heart disease, diabetes, lower back pain, stroke, and several types of cancer. Although some people consider cellulite largely a cosmetic concern, it may be an indication of various health risks related to excess body fat.

With so much more fat and so much less muscle, the appearance of cellulite is almost inevitable. Keep in mind that most women have most of their fat storage in areas below the waist, typically in their hips and thighs. Add to this the fact that muscle is lost when and where it is not used. Because sitting occupies so much time in our sedentary society, the hip and thigh muscles are among the first to atrophy.

When an area has too little muscle and too much fat, the underlying foundation loses its firmness and the skin assumes the loose and lumpy appearance referred to as cellulite. Although the overwhelming response to the cellulite problem is dieting, this single-pronged approach cannot successfully address a two-pronged problem.

3 | Why Dieting Doesn't Work

YOU will note that the average aging woman experiences two equally undesirable changes in body composition, namely muscle loss and fat gain. Of course, inactive women may see these changes earlier in life, starting in their late teens or twenties. Because these are two basic problems, remediation requires two specific solutions. The main reason that dieting almost always proves unsuccessful is because it addresses only one of the basic problems: fat gain. Unfortunately, dieting actually exacerbates the other problem, muscle loss, making the cellulite as well as the imbalance between fat and muscle worse than before dieting.

Because most people do not enjoy dieting, they try to lose their excess body fat as quickly as possible. Therefore, they follow very low-calorie diets that expedite a more rapid weight reduction. However, when food energy is in short supply, our bodies break down muscle tissue as well as utilize stored fat to make up the difference. Consequently, about 25 percent of the body weight lost on very low-calorie diets is muscle.

For example, if our average 50-year-old woman loses 30 pounds of body weight, she will again weigh 126 pounds (see Figure 2.1 in Chapter Two). However, her weight loss actually represents 22.5 pounds less fat and 7.5 pounds less muscle. Unlike her commendable body composition when she was 20 years old (30 pounds of fat and 45 pounds of muscle), her 126 pounds now consists of 52.5 pounds of fat and 22.5 pounds of muscle. Although she weighs the same on the bathroom scale, she actually has 22.5 pounds more fat (30 pounds vs. 52.5 pounds) and 22.5 pounds less muscle (45 pounds vs. 22.5 pounds).

With only half of her original muscle tissue, our well-intentioned 50-year-old woman now has an extremely low resting metabolism. Assuming that every pound of muscle tissue requires at least 30 calories a day for resting function, 22.5 pounds less muscle means almost 700 fewer calories a day for resting metabolism at age 50 than at age 20. That amount of calorie limitation may be possible for a brief period of dieting, but it can't be maintained for long. Consequently, when she resumes more normal eating patterns, the food portions that previously maintained her body weight will now produce consistent weight gain. Unfortunately, she faces an unfair and puzzling predicament. She can't continue the very-low-calorie diet indefinitely, and she can't eat normally without gaining body fat.

This frustrating situation is responsible for 95 percent of all dieters regaining all the weight they lost within one year after discontinuing their diet program. At best, dieting alone provides only a temporary weight loss that presents more problems than it seems to solve. So if dieting doesn't work, what does?

Although dieting can be an effective means for reducing body fat, it does not replace lost muscle. Dieting can help solve one body composition problem (too much fat), but it actually intensifies the other problem (too little muscle). Productive and permanent improvement in body composition can only be attained when strength training is part of the repackaging process.

4 | Understanding Strength Training

MOST people associate strength training with building up rather than trimming down. They have heard that strength training builds muscle and increases body weight, whereas endurance exercise burns calories and decreases body weight. Of course, overweight individuals have no interest in increasing their body weight. So if they do choose to exercise, it is typically some form of aerobic activity, such as walking, cycling, stepping, or dancing. These physical activities definitely burn calories and result in reduced body fat, as long as the total number of calories used exceeds the total number of calories consumed.

Unfortunately, endurance exercise does not replace lost muscle, nor does it prevent the muscle atrophy associated with the aging process. Like dieting, aerobic activity is helpful for reducing body fat, but it does not have a positive effect on muscle maintenance, which is most useful for permanent weight management.

This is why strength training is essential for improving body composition and enhancing physical appearance. Without question, strength training is the most important ingredient in the cellulite solution. As you already know, strength training is the only means for replacing your lost muscle and recharging your resting metabolism. According to several research studies, every pound of muscle that you add through strength exercise increases your resting metabolic rate by 30 to 40 calories per day. Of course, more muscle means more calories burned during physical activity as well as at rest.

A previously sedentary adult can expect to replace 2 to 3 pounds of muscle tissue after two to three months of regular strength training. Consider the results of a classic study conducted a few years ago at Tufts University in Boston.

Twelve inactive men and women were housed in a dormitory for three months. They lived essentially sedentary lifestyles, with the exception of three relatively brief strength training sessions per week. After 12 weeks, the subjects added 3 pounds of lean (muscle) weight and lost 4 pounds of fat weight. The 3-pound muscle gain produced a 7 percent increase in their resting metabolic rate (108 more calories per day) and a 15 percent increase in their total energy requirement (370 more calories per day).

You may wonder how three standard strength training sessions per week can generate such a large increase in overall calorie utilization. Strength training has a threefold effect on energy use and is actually far more beneficial for fat loss than an equal period of endurance exercise.

First, a 30-minute circuit-style strength workout uses about 240 calories during the actual training session. This generates roughly the same number of calories required for a 30-minute walk, jog, or cycle.

Second, because strength exercise is relatively intense anaerobic activity, your metabolism remains elevated for several hours after the training session. Research indicates that you might burn 25 percent as many calories as your workout energy expenditure during the following two hours. That is between the 30-minute strength workout (240 calories) and the two-hour post-exercise period (60 calories), your net energy utilization is 300 calories.

Third, assuming that after three months of strength training, you add 3 pounds of muscle, you will burn an extra 100 calories a day at rest just to maintain your new muscle tissue.

Calorie Cost of Strength Exercise	Each Training Day
30-minute exercise circuit	240 calories/session
2-hour post-exercise period	60 calories/session
3 lbs. new muscle	100 calories/day
Total calorie cost per training day	400 calories/day

Let's do the calorie calculations on a weekly basis. After three months of training, you use 100 more calories every day, totaling 700 calories per week. On your three strength training days, you burn 300 more calories, totalling about 900 calories per week. Adding these together, your three-day-per-week strength training program accounts for approximately 1,600 more calories per week than staying sedentary and about 800 more calories per week than a three-day-per-week endurance exercise program of equal duration (30 minutes per session).

Of course, we have nothing against endurance exercise and strongly recommend its inclusion in any weight loss program. However, our research clearly indicates that endurance exercise in combination with strength training is far superior to endurance exercise alone.

In one study, 72 men and women exercised 30 minutes a day, three days a week, for a period of eight weeks. All the subjects were given heart-healthy dietary guidelines for reducing fat weight in a safe and sensible manner.

As presented in Table 4.1, the 22 participants who did only endurance exercise (30 minutes of stationary cycling) lost 4 pounds of fat but added 0 pounds of muscle, for a 4-pound reduction in body weight and a 4-pound improvement in body composition. Compare these good results with the superior results attained by the 50 subjects who performed both endurance exercise and strength training (15 minutes of stationary cycling plus seven Nautilus machines). These individuals concurrently lost 10 pounds of fat and added 2 pounds of muscle, for an 8-pound reduction in body weight and a 12-pound improvement in body composition and physical appearance.

These results attest to the advantages of a combination weight management program that includes a sensible nutrition plan, endurance exercise, and strength training. Several follow-up studies produced strikingly similar results. Table 4.2 presents the cumulative findings from 313 men and women who completed an eight-week fitness program that combined general dietary guidelines, endurance exercise, and strength training. On average, these individuals lost 8 pounds of fat and added 3 pounds of muscle, for a 5-pound reduction in body weight and an 11-pound improvement in body composition and physical appearance.

Keep in mind that the change in body weight is not nearly as important as the change in body composition. While a 5-pound reduction in body weight might not seem that impressive, an 11-pound improvement in body composition is a major accomplishment. Remember, we are dealing with a two-part problem (too little muscle and too much fat), and we need a two-part solution (more muscle and less fat).

According to the U.S. Public Health Service, we should not lose more than 1 pound per week if we expect to prevent the fat from returning. This is exactly what our program participants averaged, an 8-pound fat loss in eight weeks of training. Even more important for physical fitness, metabolic function, and personal appearance, our subjects added 3 pounds of calorie-burning muscle tissue. No wonder more than 90 percent of the program graduates reported high satisfaction with the strength exercises and committed to continue their strength workouts.

Body composition can be measured by skinfold calipers or other means at most YMCAs and fitness facilities. We recommend a body composition assessment before and after your cellulite reduction program to see how much fat you

Table 4.1

Body composition changes for 72 men and women who did endurance exercise alone (22 participants) or endurance exercise and strength training (50 participants). All participants did three 30-minute workouts per week for eight weeks.

Group	Change in Body Weight	Change in Fat Weight	Change in Muscle Weight	Change in Body Composition
Endurance exercise only (30 min.)	−4.0 lbs	−4.0 lbs	0 lbs	4.0 lbs
Endurance and strength exercise (15 min. each)	−8.0 lbs	−10.0 lbs	+2.0 lbs	12.0 lbs

Table 4.2

Cumulative findings from 313 men and women who completed an eight-week fitness program consisting of endurance exercise and strength training.

Group	Change in Body Weight	Change in Fat Weight	Change in Muscle Weight	Change in Body Composition
A (50)	−8.0 lbs	−10.0 lbs	+2.0 lbs	12.0 lbs
B (61)	−3.0 lbs	−6.0 lbs	+3.0 lbs	9.0 lbs
C (90)	−6.0 lbs	−9.5 lbs	+3.5 lbs	13.0 lbs
D (81)	−4.5 lbs	−7.5 lbs	+3.0 lbs	10.5 lbs
E (31)	−1.5 lbs	−5.0 lbs	+3.5 lbs	8.5 lbs
Total (313)	**−5.0 lbs**	**−8.0 lbs**	**+3.0 lbs**	**11.0 lbs**

lost and how much muscle you replaced. Remember, a 6-pound weight loss could actually represent 9 pounds less fat and 3 pounds more muscle for a 12-pound improvement in your body composition and physical appearance.

Summary

Always remember that muscle is good and that rebuilding muscle tissue makes you look better, feel better, and function better. Just as important, adding muscle increases your metabolism so you burn more calories all day long. After two to three months of regular strength exercise, you should replace 2 to 3 pounds of muscle, which can raise your metabolic rate up to 7 percent. Of course, strength exercise is vigorous physical activity that burns lots of calories during your training session and even for a couple hours after your workout. Research indicates that a basic program of strength and endurance exercise, along with sensible eating, can replace 3 pounds of muscle and reduce 8 pounds of fat after just eight weeks of training.

5 | General Strength Training Guidelines

OUR research has shown the benefits of strength training for weight loss and better body composition. In order to begin your safe, effective, and efficient program of strength exercise, here are the basic recommendations you should follow for best results.

Principle of Progression: Resistance and Repetitions

Perhaps the most practical definition of strength training is progressive resistance exercise. In other words, to develop more strength and muscle tissue, you must gradually increase your exercise weightloads. For example, let's assume you can presently lift 50 pounds 15 times in the leg extension exercise. Repeating this workout (15 repetitions with 50 pounds) will maintain your leg extension strength but will not develop stronger quadriceps muscles. Increasing the number of repetitions to 16, 17, 18, and so on has some strength-building benefit, but at this point, adding exercise repetitions is not nearly as productive as adding exercise resistance. While doing more repetitions increases the exercise duration, using more resistance (heavier weightloads) increases the exercise intensity, which is much more effective for muscle development.

How do you determine an appropriate resistance level and repetition range for making progressive strength improvements? The key factor is to complete each set of strength exercise within the anaerobic energy system. For most practical purposes, your anaerobic energy system enables you to perform between 30 and 90 seconds of continuous, high-effort exercise. Therefore, you want to use enough resistance to fatigue your target muscle group within that time frame.

If you perform your exercise repetitions in a slow and controlled manner (about six seconds each), your effective repetition range encompasses 5 to 15 repetitions per set. Although our research indicates that training anywhere within this range will increase your muscle strength, we recommend using 10 to 15 repetitions per set. Exercising at the higher end of the repetition range permits a greater training volume and requires more energy expenditure.

For example, if you perform 5 repetitions with 100 pounds, you will do 500 pounds of work in about 30 seconds. On the other hand, if you complete 15 repetitions with 70 pounds, you will do 1,050 pounds of work in about 90 seconds. Both training protocols provide high-effort anaerobic exercise, and both are effective for increasing your muscle strength. However, the higher repetition program enables you to accomplish twice as much total work, which utilizes twice as many calories.

Implementing the principle of progressive resistance means adding more weight whenever you complete 15 repetitions in good form. For example, if you perform 15 repetitions with 70 pounds today, you should increase the resistance about 5 percent (3 to 4 pounds) at your next workout. The heavier weightload may reduce your repetitions to 12 or 13, which is a normal response. Stay with this resistance until you can again complete 15 good repetitions, then increase the weightload by another 5 percent.

> RECOMMENDATION: Use a resistance that you can perform for at least 10 repetitions. When you can complete 15 repetitions, add about 5 percent more resistance (typically 1 to 5 pounds, depending on your training weightload).

Principle of Progression: Sets

Another aspect of progressive strength training is the number of sets you perform each exercise. Let's say you do 15 Leg Extensions with 60 pounds, rest a minute, then do 15 Leg Curls with 45 pounds. You have performed each exercise for one set of 15 repetitions. This type of strength training is called circuit training because you complete one set of each exercise in the circuit with a brief rest between stations.

Research has demonstrated that single-set circuit training is as effective as multiple-set workouts for developing muscle strength. Clearly, single-set exercise sessions are more time-efficient than multiple-set exercise sessions. These positive features (minimum time and maximum results) make single-set strength training ideal for beginning exercisers.

However, as you become more proficient at strength training, you may choose to do two or three sets of each exercise. The main disadvantage of multiple-set training is longer workouts for essentially the same rate of strength development. The main advantage of multiple-set training is greater training volume, which results in more energy expenditure.

If you enjoy your strength workouts and have plenty of training time, you may gradually progress to a second or even a third set of each exercise. Just be careful not to do too much too soon, to reduce the risk of overtraining. When performing multiple sets, rest about two minutes between each set to replenish your muscle energy stores.

Based on our research studies and professional experience, we favor single-set training, especially if your workouts include several strength exercises. For example, if you are doing only five exercises targeting your hips and thighs, you would need 30 minutes to complete a two-set strength workout, which is a reasonable time commitment. However, if you were doing 10 exercises for total body training, you would need more than 90 minutes to complete a three-set strength workout, which may be impractical for many people. Compare this to a 10-exercise single-set strength workout that requires only 25 minutes for completion. Because time is a limiting factor for most exercisers, we generally recommend that you do one good set of each strength exercise.

> **RECOMMENDATION:** Perform one good set of each strength exercise for the best combination of training effectiveness and time efficiency.

Single-set strength training is particularly productive when you perform as many repetitions as possible to the point of muscle fatigue. That is, you don't stop the exercise set until your target muscles can no longer lift the weightload with proper technique.

However, if you desire even greater strength-building stimulus, you may progress to a higher-intensity workout technique known as breakdown training. Breakdown training is an efficient means for eliciting more muscle effort, thereby enhancing strength development.

As an example of breakdown training, let's say you can complete 12 good leg presses with 200 pounds. At the point when you can no longer lift this weightload, immediately reduce the resistance by about 10 percent (180 pounds). Without resting, perform as many additional repetitions as possible with the lighter weightload. Typically, you will be able to do two to five more repetitions with the reduced resistance before reaching a second level of muscle fatigue. These few post-fatigue repetitions have a significant impact on muscle development, with up to 40 percent greater strength gains than standard training.

Of course, it is not necessary to progress to breakdown training, especially if you find standard strength exercise sufficiently challenging. However, this is a time-efficient means for increasing the intensity of each exercise set should you desire to do so. You should be encouraged to know that harder training does not necessarily require longer exercise sessions.

> RECOMMENDATION: One means for increasing the intensity of your exercise set is to perform breakdown training. Upon completing as many repetitions as possible with your standard weightload, reduce the resistance by about 10 percent and perform a few additional repetitions to reach a second level of muscle fatigue.

Principle of Muscle Activation

Much of the effectiveness of a strength training program is related to your exercise technique. You can train in a controlled manner that maximizes the muscle stimulus of each repetition, or you can train in a sloppy manner that minimizes the muscle stimulus of each repetition. Worse yet, training with poor exercise technique can cause injuries to your musculoskeletal system and should always be avoided.

Proper strength training technique consists of three critical components: body posture, movement speed, and movement range. As simple as it may seem, these are the essential factors for safe and effective strength exercise. Let's take a closer look at each aspect of proper form and productive strength training.

Body Posture

Performing each exercise with proper posture provides two important benefits. First, when training with good posture, your body segments are properly aligned to maximize your muscular ability and to minimize your injury risk. That is, correct posture enables you to better execute the exercise movement and better emphasize the target muscle groups.

Second, maintaining good posture throughout each exercise set requires greater energy expenditure, thereby increasing the calorie cost of your strength training session. We have also noticed that people who emphasize body position during their workouts are more attentive to posture throughout the day, whether sitting, standing, or walking. Without question, proper body positioning makes your exercise efforts more productive and enhances your physical appearance inside and outside the fitness facility.

RECOMMENDATION: Stress good posture and proper body alignment throughout every strength exercise.

Movement Speed

In our opinion, the most critical factor for safe and productive strength training is using controlled movement speed. Slow exercise speeds place less stress on your joints and provide more tension for your muscles, both of which are desirable. Conversely, fast exercise speeds place more stress on your joints and provide less tension for your muscles, both of which are undesirable.

Lifting and lowering weights quickly is similar to throwing and catching a heavy object. Starting and stopping a fast-moving resistance typically requires too much force for safe exercise experiences. In addition, explosive actions employ momentum throughout most of the movement range, which reduces the training effect on the target muscles. In other words, fast movement speeds are associated with more injury risk and less strength stimulus. So don't be tempted to try rapid repetitions, even if other exercisers train in this manner. If you exercise control, your results will inevitably exceed those who train in an explosive manner. That is, controlled exercise usually results in strength progression for longer periods of time than does momentum-assisted training at fast speeds.

Our suggested exercise speed is six seconds per repetition, which requires one minute for a set of 10 repetitions and 90 seconds for a set of 15 repetitions. These slower-speed repetitions permit more muscle tension and more muscle force, both of which enhance strength development.

You can lower almost 50 percent more weight than you can lift. For this reason, we recommend that you perform each lifting movement in two seconds and each lowering movement in four seconds. By taking twice as long on your lowering movements, the resistance that would otherwise feel too light during this phase requires plenty of effort and provides significant muscle stimulus.

The main consideration with training speed is to be in complete control of the resistance throughout every exercise repetition. Remember, the purpose of strength training is to use muscle, rather than momentum, for lifting and lowering appropriate weightloads. We believe that slow exercise speeds are synonymous with safe, sensible, and successful strength workouts.

RECOMMENDATION: Perform every exercise repetition in a slow and controlled manner. Take two seconds for each lifting movement and four seconds for each lowering movement.

Movement Range

To develop strength throughout the full range of joint movement, you must exercise the target muscles from a moderately stretched position to a fully contracted position. In other words, to develop full-range strength, you must perform full-range exercise. Of course, you should never move the resistance into painful positions. However, you will achieve better results if you train the full, pain-free, range of every exercise.

When you combine slow movement speed and full movement range, you have an unbeatable combination for maximizing the strength-building benefit of every exercise repetition. Additionally, this strict approach to strength training minimizes your risk of injury, making for safe and productive exercise experiences.

> RECOMMENDATION: **Perform every exercise repetition through a full range of pain-free movement, from a moderately stretched position to a fully contracted position.**

Principle of Proper Breathing

You might not think about your breathing pattern when you perform strength exercise, but the natural tendency is to hold your breath during the moments of most exertion. Unfortunately, breath-holding invariably increases your blood pressure response to strength training and should definitely be avoided.

With proper breathing, your blood pressure responds similarly to both strength training and endurance exercise, and the end result is typically a reduction in your resting blood pressure. The proper breathing during strength exercise is to exhale throughout each lifting movement and inhale throughout each lowering movement. This breathing technique is easy to learn (think up and out), and results in lower exercise blood pressure responses.

As you practice this breathing pattern, you should find that your exercise repetitions are easier to perform and that you recover more quickly at the end of your exercise set. Make every effort to breathe out during your two-second lifting movements and to breathe in during your four-second lowering movements.

> **RECOMMENDATION:** Exhale throughout the lifting phase (two seconds) and inhale throughout the lowering phase (four seconds) of every exercise repetition. Never hold your breath when strength training.

Principle of Muscle Balance

The cellulite reduction program targets the muscles of the hips and thighs. These muscles are addressed in a balanced manner, with the Leg Extension exercise for the front thigh, the Leg Curl exercise for the rear thigh, the Hip Adduction exercise for the inner thigh, the Hip Abduction exercise for the outer thigh, and the Leg Press exercise that works most of the hip and thigh muscles simultaneously.

A well-balanced strength training program includes all the body's major muscle groups. To accomplish this, we add two exercises for the midsection muscles and three exercises for the upper body muscles. These are balanced in the following manner: the Abdominal Curl for the front midsection muscles; the Low Back Extension for the rear midsection muscles; the Bench Press for the chest and rear arm muscles; the Seated Row for the upper back and front arm muscles; and the Overhead Press for the shoulder and rear arm muscles.

Although it is tempting to assign similar weightloads to opposing muscle groups, this is not always advisable. For example, you have five muscles in your Hip Adductor group (inner thigh), but only two muscles in your Hip Abductor group (outer thigh). Consequently, you can use much more resistance in the Hip Adduction exercise than in the Hip Abduction exercise. To attain the most strength benefit and to maintain the best muscle balance, use a resistance that permits 10 to 15 repetitions for each exercise.

> RECOMMENDATION: Select strength exercises that address all the major muscle groups, for example, five exercises for the lower body and five exercises for the upper body/midsection.

Design your strength training program to perform exercises for your larger muscle groups followed by exercises for your smaller muscle groups. Generally speaking, begin with the leg exercises, proceed to the upper body exercises, and finish with the midsection exercises. Placing the midsection exercises at the end of the workout prevents these important posture and stabilization muscles from fatiguing prematurely, which could reduce the effectiveness of other exercises.

We also recommend pairing the exercises for opposite joint actions. For example, pair the Leg Extension and Leg Curl exercises, the Hip Adduction and Hip Abduction exercises, the Abdominal Curl and Low Back Extension exercises, and the Bench Press and Seated Row exercises. The Leg Press may be the last lower body exercise, and the Overhead Press may be the final upper body exercise.

Tables 5.1 and 5.2 present our recommended strength exercises, the target muscle groups, and the preferred order of performance when using either weight-stack machines or free weights. Given about 90 seconds to perform each exercise and about a minute break between exercises, this 10-station workout should take less than 25 minutes.

> RECOMMENDATION: Perform strength exercises in order from larger to smaller muscle groups, pairing exercises that use opposite joint actions.

Table 5.1

Recommended strength exercises, target muscle groups, and preferred order of performance using weightstack machines.

Exercise Order Machines	Target Muscle Groups
Leg extension machine	Quadriceps (front thigh)
Leg curl machine	Hamstrings (rear thigh)
Hip adduction machine	Hip adductors (inner thigh)
Hip abduction machine	Hip abductors (outer thigh)
Leg press machine	Quadriceps (front thigh), hamstrings (rear thigh), and gluteals (buttocks)
Bench press machine	Pectoralis major (chest) and triceps (rear arm)
Seated row machine	Latissimus dorsi (upper back) and biceps (front arm)
Overhead press machine	Deltoids (shoulders) and triceps (rear arm)
Low back extension	Erector spinae (rear midsection)
Abdominal curl machine	Rectus abdominis (front midsection)

Table 5.2

Recommended strength exercises, target muscle groups, and preferred order of performance using free weights, elastic bands, and body weight.

Exercise Order Free Weights	Target Muscle Groups
Dumbbell Squat	Quadriceps (front thigh), hamstrings (rear thigh), and gluteals (buttocks)
Dumbbell Lunge	Quadriceps (front thigh), hamstrings (rear thigh), and gluteals (buttocks)
Dumbbell Step-Up	Quadriceps (front thigh), hamstrings (rear thigh), and gluteals (buttocks)
Band Hip Adduction	Hip adductors (inner thigh)
Band Hip Abduction	Hip abductors (outer thigh)
Dumbbell Bench Press	Pectoralis major (chest) and triceps (rear arm)
Dumbbell Bent Row	Latissimus dorsi (upper back) and biceps (front arm)
Dumbbell Overhead Press	Deltoids (shoulders) and triceps (rear arm)
Body Weight Trunk Extension	Erector spinae (rear midsection)
Body Weight Trunk Curl	Rectus abdominis (front midsection)

Principle of Muscle Recovery

You now have all the components necessary for an efficient exercise session that effectively stimulates muscle development. However, for a strength workout to produce the desired results, it must be followed by a nontraining period that permits the muscles to fully recover and reach higher strength levels.

Your muscles actually become weaker during a set of high-effort strength exercises. During the following recovery period, they gradually gain strength and become slightly stronger than before. Although optimum recovery periods vary among individual exercisers, most people attain peak muscle strength approximately two days after their last exercise session.

Ideally, each strength workout should be taken at the highest point of your recovery process, which is typically achieved by an every-other-day training schedule. We recommend strength training on Mondays, Wednesdays, and Fridays with an extra recovery day during the weekends. This three-day-per-week training schedule has produced excellent results for the participants in our cellulite reduction research programs.

We realize that some people cannot commit to three training sessions every week. Fortunately, our studies have shown 75 to 85 percent as much benefit from two weekly strength workouts. Although we prefer an every-other-day training program, two weekly strength workouts should be sufficient for significant improvements in your cellulite situation.

> RECOMMENDATION: Perform two or three evenly spaced strength training sessions per week, such as a Monday-Wednesday-Friday schedule or a Monday and Thursday schedule.

Summary of Strength Training Guidelines

Our studies suggest that strength exercise is the first step in a successful cellulite reduction program. Regaining firm, fit, and attractive muscles and recharging your metabolism are key factors in reducing fat stores and reshaping your hips and thighs, as well as your entire body. The following recommendations should ensure safe, effective, and efficient strength training experiences that enable you to look better, feel better, and function better.

one | **RECOMMENDATION:**

RESISTANCE AND REPETITIONS: Use a resistance you can perform for at least 10 repetitions. When you can complete 15 repetitions, add about 5 percent more resistance.

Note: Be sure to use proper exercise technique on every repetition.

two | **RECOMMENDATION:**

SETS: Perform one good set of each strength exercise for the best combination of training effectiveness and time efficiency.

Note: Use single-set exercise sessions to reduce the risk of overtraining.

three | **RECOMMENDATION:**

HIGHER INTENSITY: Perform breakdown training to increase the intensity of your exercise set. Upon completing as many repetitions as possible with your standard weightload, reduce the resistance by about 10 percent and perform a few additional repetitions to reach a second level of muscle fatigue.

Note: Use breakdown training as a time-efficient means for extending your exercise set and eliciting greater strength gains.

four | **RECOMMENDATION:**

BODY POSTURE: Use good posture and proper body alignment throughout every strength exercise.

Note: Try to sit tall and stand tall when strength training.

five | **RECOMMENDATION:**

MOVEMENT SPEED: Perform every exercise repetition in a slow and controlled manner. Take two seconds for each lifting movement and four seconds for each lowering movement.

Note: Avoid fast exercise speeds that decrease your strength benefits and increase your injury risks.

six | **RECOMMENDATION:**

MOVEMENT RANGE: Perform every exercise repetition through a full range of pain-free movement, from a moderately stretched position to a fully contracted position.

Note: Always adjust your exercise movements to avoid joint discomfort.

seven | **RECOMMENDATION:**

PROPER BREATHING: Exhale throughout the lifting phase (two seconds) and inhale throughout the lowering phase (four seconds) of every exercise repetition.

Note: Never hold your breath when strength training.

eight **RECOMMENDATION:**

MUSCLE BALANCE: Select strength exercises that address all the major muscle groups, for example, five exercises for the lower body and five exercises for the upper body/midsection.

Note: Always choose a total body strength training program over a spot exercise plan.

nine **RECOMMENDATION:**

EXERCISE SEQUENCE: Perform strength exercises in order from larger to smaller muscle groups, pairing exercises that use opposite joint actions.

Note: Use a recommended exercise sequence to enhance the strength training process.

ten **RECOMMENDATION:**

MUSCLE RECOVERY: Perform two or three evenly spaced strength training sessions per week, such as a Monday-Wednesday-Friday schedule or a Monday and Thursday schedule.

Note: Avoid strength exercise on consecutive days, as this does not permit sufficient time for muscle building.

6 | Specific Strength Training Exercises

GENERALLY speaking, you can perform strength exercises with free weights (barbells and dumbbells) or machines, and the choice is largely a matter of personal preference. Advantages of free weights include lower equipment costs, at-home training, more workout versatility, and greater freedom of exercise. The disadvantages include more training experience, greater exercise skill, and higher risk of injury.

Advantages of machines include supportive structure, relatively fixed movement patterns, enhanced muscle isolation, reduced injury risk, and training efficiency. The disadvantages include higher equipment cost, greater space requirements, and more challenging fit for small women.

If you have access to a well-equipped fitness facility, we recommend a 10-machine training program with five specific exercises for your hips and thighs and five additional exercises for your upper body and midsection. The exercises are the leg extension, leg curl, hip adduction, hip abduction, leg press, bench press, seated row, overhead press, low back extension, and abdominal curl. Be sure to ask a fitness instructor how to properly use each machine, as the procedures may vary among different models/manufacturers.

If you choose to train at home, we recommend a combination of dumbbell, elastic band, and body weight exercises that address the same major muscle groups in a slightly different manner. These exercises are dumbbell squats, dumbbell lunges, dumbbell step-ups, band hip adductions, band hip abductions, dumbbell bench presses, dumbbell bent rows, dumbbell overhead presses, body weight trunk extensions, and body weight trunk curls.

This chapter presents explanations and illustrations of all the machine and free-weight exercises so you can perform the desired movement patterns safely and effectively. Remember to use slow movement speeds and full movement range on every exercise repetition. We advise taking two full seconds to lift the weight and four full seconds to lower the weight. Be sure to breathe continuously, exhaling during each lifting phase and inhaling during each lowering phase. Select a resistance that enables you to complete one set of 10 to 15 repetitions in good form. Upon progressing to 15 repetitions, add about 5 percent more resistance for your next training session. Once you become familiar with the strength training procedures, the 10-exercise strength workout should take no more than 25 minutes for completion.

Equipment You Will Need
For Home Strength Training

To train at home, you will need a pair of adjustable dumbbells or a few sets of fixed-weight dumbbells, typically ranging from 3 to 20 pounds. You will use lighter dumbbells for upper body exercises and heavier dumbbells for leg exercises. We suggest the following dumbbell sets based on your present level of strength fitness.

STRENGTH LEVEL	DUMBBELL SETS
Low	3 lbs, 5 lbs, 8 lbs, 10 lbs, 12 lbs
Medium	5 lbs, 8 lbs, 10 lbs, 12 lbs, 15 lbs
High	8 lbs, 10 lbs, 12 lbs, 15 lbs, 20 lbs

You will also need elastic exercise bands for two leg exercises. We recommend exercise bands with handles for safety and simplicity. Exercise bands come in different resistance levels designated by different colors. You will use less resistance on the hip abduction exercise than on the hip adduction exercise, so a full set of exercise bands may be useful.

Most sporting goods stores sell dumbbells and exercise bands. If those in your area do not, consider the following sources for quality resistance equipment.

York Barbell Company:
Phone: 800-358-9675   Web: *yorkbarbell.com*

SPRI Products, Inc.:
Phone: 800-222-7774   Web: *spriproducts.com*

Leg Extension

muscles	Front thighs (quadriceps)
starting position	Sit on seat with back against seatback, hands on handles, and ankles behind ankle pad.
movement	Bring legs from a right angle to a straight line by extending knees.
ending position	Legs should be straight, approximately parallel to the floor.
key points	▪ Keep ankles at right angles throughout exercise. ▪ Do not lean forward during the lifting action. ▪ Exhale as you lift the weightstack in two seconds, and inhale as you lower the weightstack in four seconds.

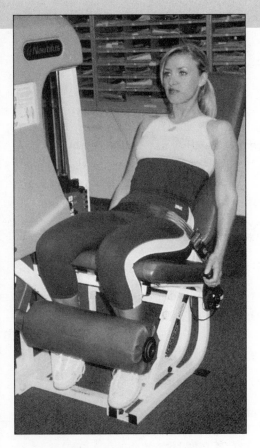

Leg Extension—Start

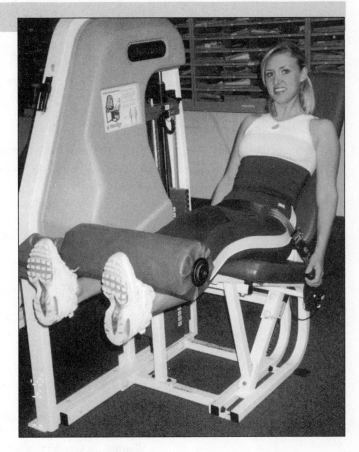

Leg Extension—Finish

Seated Leg Curl

muscles	Rear thighs (hamstrings)
starting position	Sit on seat with back against seatback, hands on handles, and legs between shin and ankle pads.
movement	Bring heels toward buttocks by flexing knees.
ending position	Heels should be as close as possible to seat bottom with rear thigh muscles fully contracted.
key points	• Keep ankles at right angles throughout exercise. • Do not arch your back during the lifting action. • Exhale as you lift the weightstack in two seconds, and inhale as you lower the weightstack in four seconds.

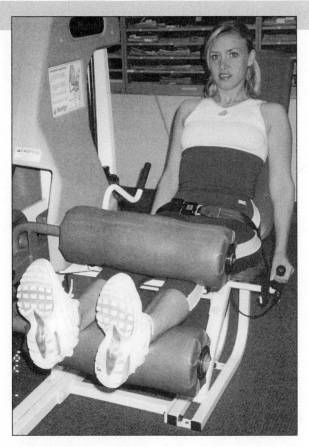

Seated Leg Curl—Start

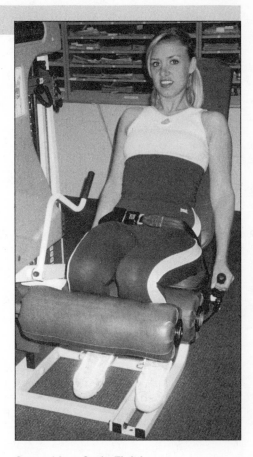

Seated Leg Curl—Finish

Hip Adduction

muscles

Inner thighs (hip adductors)

starting position

Sit on seat with back against seatback, hands on handles, and legs outside movement pads, spread comfortably apart.

movement

Bring thighs together.

ending position

Thighs should be as close together as possible.

key points

- Apply muscle force against the thigh movement pads rather than the ankle pads.

- Exhale as you lift the weightstack in two seconds, and inhale as you lower the weightstack in four seconds.

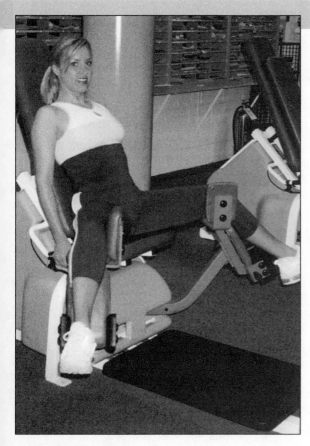

Hip Adduction—Start

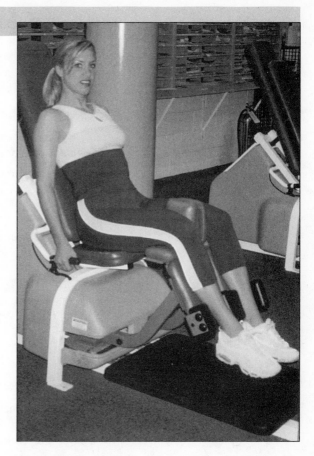

Hip Adduction—Finish

Hip Abduction

muscles

Outer thighs (hip abductors)

starting position

Sit on seat with back against seatback, hands on handles, and legs inside movement pads, thighs together.

movement

Spread thighs apart.

ending position

Thighs should be spread as far apart as possible without discomfort.

key points

- Apply muscle force through the thigh movement pads rather than the ankle pads.

- Do not arch your lower back during the lifting action.

- Exhale as you lift the weightstack in two seconds, and inhale as you lower the weightstack in four seconds.

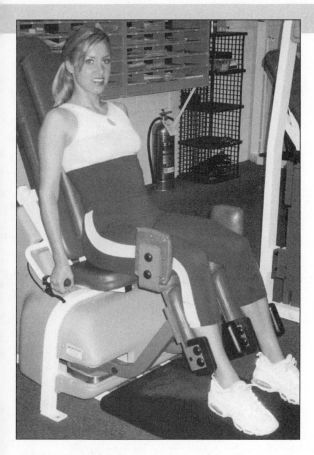

Hip Abduction—Start

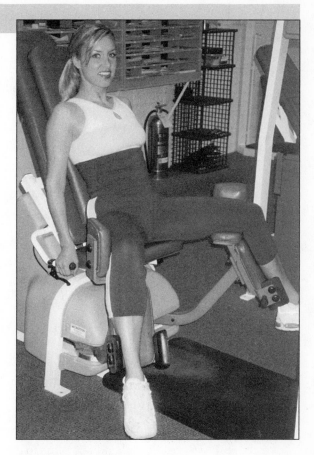

Hip Abduction—Finish

Leg Press

muscles

Front thighs (quadriceps)
Rear thighs (hamstrings)
Buttocks (gluteals)

starting position

Sit on seat with back against seatback, feet equally spaced on foot plate, and knees at right angles.

movement

Push feet forward until legs are almost straight with knees just slightly bent.

ending position

Legs should be almost straight with knees close to full extension but not locked out.

key points

- Use arms to assist with the first repetition by pushing your thighs forward if necessary.

- Keep ankles, knees, and hips equally spaced and in line throughout exercise.

- Stop just short of knee lockout on every repetition.

- Exhale as you lift the weightstack in two seconds, and inhale as you lower the weightstack in four seconds.

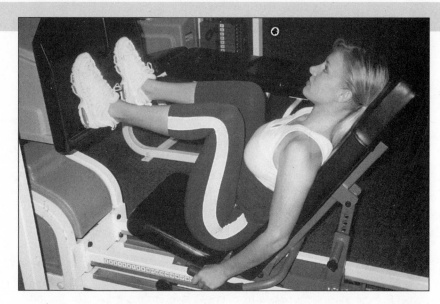

Leg Press—Start

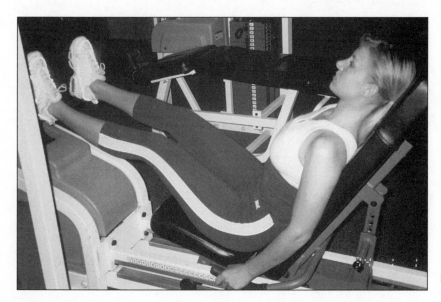

Leg Press—Finish

Bench Press

muscles

Chest (pectoralis major)

Shoulders (anterior deltoid)

Rear arms (triceps)

starting position

Lie face-up on bench with feet on floor or step and hands on handles in line with broadest area of chest and slightly more than shoulder width apart.

movement

Push handles upward from chest level until arms are extended above chest.

ending position

Arms should be fully extended above thickest area of chest.

key points

- Keep hips and head on bench at all times.

- Keep wrists firm and in line with forearms throughout exercise.

- Keep elbows away from sides throughout exercise.

- Exhale as you lift the weightstack in two seconds, and inhale as you lower the weightstack in four seconds.

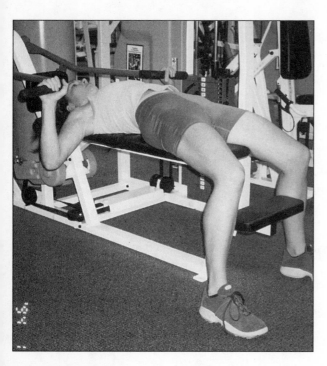

Bench Press—Start

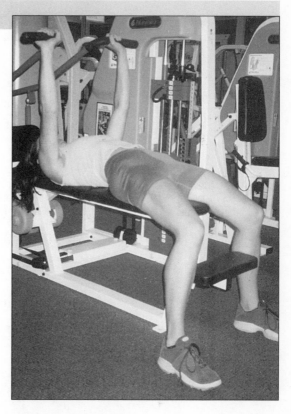

Bench Press—Finish

Compound Row

muscles
Upper back (latissimus dorsi, rhomboids, middle trapezius)
Shoulders (posterior deltoid)
Front arm (biceps)

starting position
Sit on bench with chest pressed against front restraint pad, feet on floor, and hands on upper handles with arms straight and parallel to floor.

movement
Pull handles backward from straight-arm position to chest.

ending position
Arms should be flexed with handles close to chest.

key points
- Keep head up and chest against front restraint pad throughout exercise.

- Keep wrists firm and in line with forearms throughout exercise.

- Exhale as you lift the weightstack in two seconds, and inhale as you lower the weightstack in four seconds.

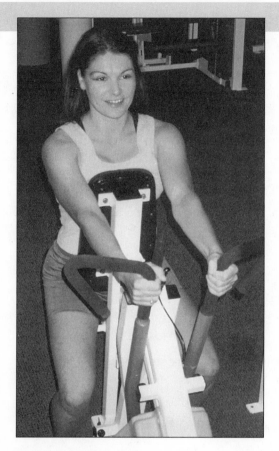

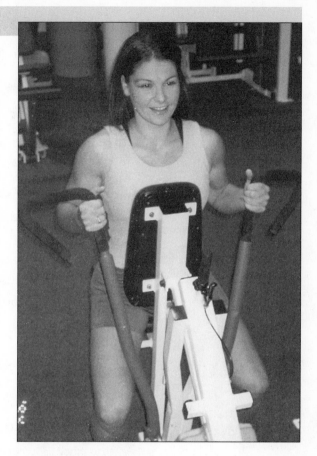

Compound Row—Start

Compound Row—Finish

Overhead Press

muscles

Shoulders (deltoids)

Rear arm (triceps)

Neck (upper trapezius)

starting position

Sit on seat with back against seatback and hands on handles just above shoulders.

movement

Push handles upward from just above shoulder level until arms are extended above shoulders.

ending position

Arms should be extended above shoulders.

key points

- Keep wrists firm and in line with forearms throughout exercise.

- Exhale as you lift the weightstack in two seconds, and inhale as you lower the weightstack in four seconds.

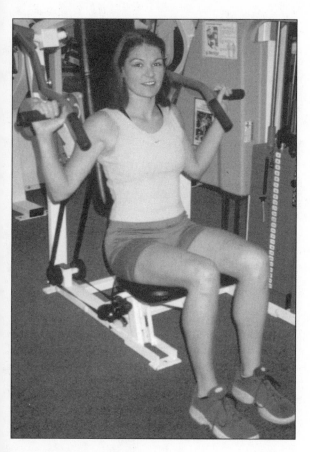

Overhead Press—Start

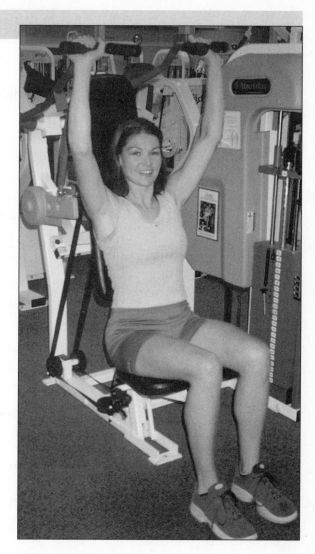

Overhead Press—Finish

Low Back Extension

muscles Lower back (erector spinae)

starting position Sit on seat with hips against seatback, feet on foot plate with knees higher than hips, seatbelts tightened securely, and arms folded across chest.

movement Move torso backward from trunk-flexed position to trunk-extended position.

ending position Torso should be extended backward as far as comfortable.

key points
- Tighten seatbelts enough to keep hips motionless throughout exercise.
- Keep head in line with spine throughout exercise.
- Exhale as you lift the weightstack in two seconds, and inhale as you lower the weightstack in four seconds.

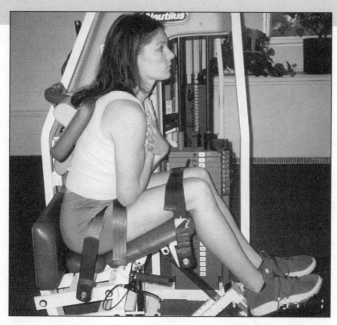

Low Back Extension—

Start

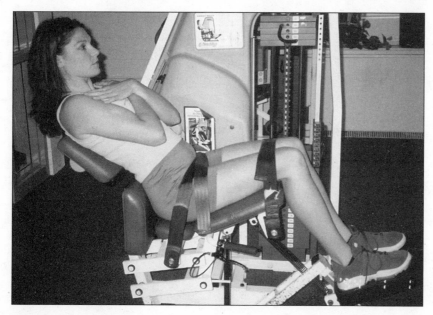

Low Back Extension—

Finish

Abdominal Curl

muscles   Midsection (rectus abdominis)

starting position   Sit on seat with hips against seatback, ankles behind ankle pads, elbows on movement pads, and hands on handles.

movement   Move torso forward from trunk-extended position to trunk-flexed position.

ending position   Torso should be flexed forward until midsection muscles are fully contracted.

key points

- Apply about 90 percent of the movement force through the elbows and about 10 percent of the movement force through the hands.

- Keep head in line with spine throughout exercise.

- Exhale as you lift the weightstack in two seconds, and inhale as you lower the weightstack in four seconds.

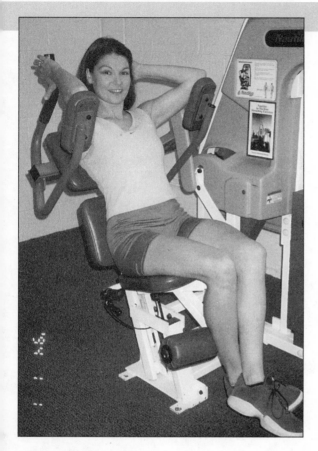

Abdominal Curl—Start

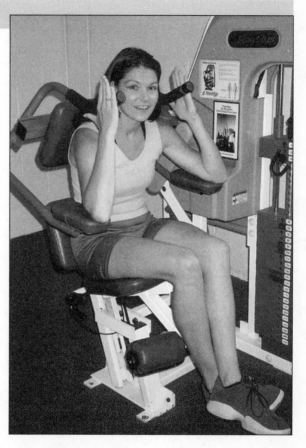

Abdominal Curl—Finish

Free-Weight Exercises
(Dumbbells, Elastic Bands, and Body Weight)

If you prefer to train at home, here are the recommended free-weight exercises using dumbbells, elastic bands, and body weight. Like the machine workout, we have five exercises for your hips and thighs and five additional exercises for your upper body and midsection. The exercises are the Dumbbell Squat, Dumbbell Lunge, Dumbbell Step-Up, Band Hip Adduction, Band Hip Abduction, Dumbbell Bench Press, Dumbbell Bent Row, Dumbbell Overhead Press, Body Weight Trunk Extension, and Body Weight Trunk Curl. Select dumbbell weightloads and elastic band resistances that fatigue your target muscles within 10 to 15 repetitions. If you cannot perform 10 repetitions, the resistance is too high, and if you can complete more than 15 repetitions, the resistance is too low. Generally speaking, the lower body dumbbell exercises may be performed with 5- to 20-pound dumbbells, depending on your personal strength level. Due to less muscle mass in the upper body, the bench press, bent row, and overhead press exercises require less resistance, typically 3- to 15-pound dumbbells based on your muscular ability and training experience. You can purchase various dumbbell sets at local sporting goods stores at reasonable prices.

Dumbbell Squat

muscles

Front thighs (quadriceps)
Rear thighs (hamstrings)
Buttocks (gluteals)

starting position

Hold the dumbbells at your sides and lower your hips downward and backward until your thighs are almost horizontal.

movement

Rise from a half-squat position to a standing position.

ending position

Legs should be extended, and back should be straight.

key points

- Keep feet about shoulder width apart throughout exercise.

- Keep torso relatively erect throughout exercise.

- Keep head in line with spine throughout exercise.

- Exhale as you ascend in two seconds, and inhale as you descend in four seconds.

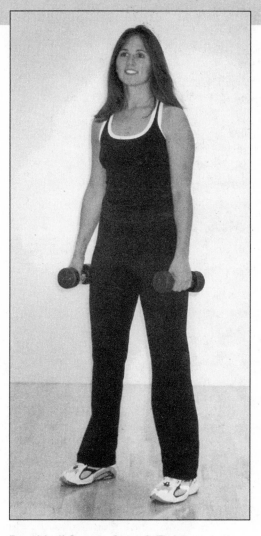

Dumbbell Squat—Start & Finish

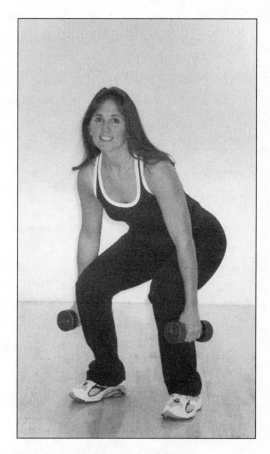

Dumbbell Squat—Down Position

Dumbbell Lunge

muscles

Front thighs (quadriceps)
Rear thighs (hamstrings)
Buttocks (gluteals)

starting position

Hold the dumbbells at your sides, and step forward so your left knee is bent 90 degrees and directly above your left foot.

movement

Rise from a lunge position to a standing position.

ending position

Legs should be extended, and back should be straight.

key points

- Step forward far enough that your knee is directly above your foot.

- Keep torso relatively erect throughout exercise.

- Keep head in line with spine throughout exercise.

- Alternate forward-stepping leg every repetition for 15 total repetitions.

- Exhale as you ascend and inhale as you descend.

note

- If the standard lunge feels uncomfortable or uncoordinated, simply do a backward lunge by stepping backward with one foot to achieve the same basic lunge position. Alternate feet with each successive backward lunge.

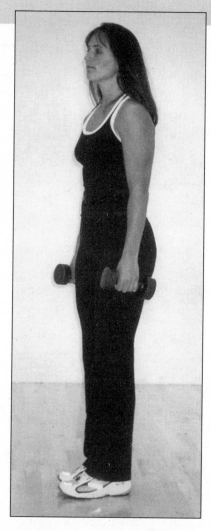

Dumbbell Lunge—Start & Finish

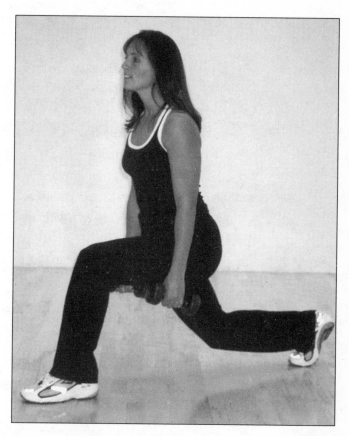

Dumbbell Lunge—Down Position

Dumbbell Step-Up

muscles

Front thighs (quadriceps)

Rear thighs (hamstrings)

Buttocks (gluteals)

starting position

Hold the dumbbells at your sides while standing on the floor and step onto a 6- to 12-inch bench or stair step one foot at a time.

movement

Step up from a floor-standing position to a bench-standing position.

ending position

Legs should be extended, and back should be straight while standing on the bench.

key points

- Place your full foot on the bench before lifting your body upward.

- Place both feet fully on the bench before lowering your body downward.

- Keep torso relatively erect throughout exercise.

- Keep head in line with spine throughout exercise.

- Alternate upward-stepping leg every repetition for 15 total repetitions.

- Keep feet relatively close to bench when stepping up and down.

- Exhale as you ascend and inhale as you descend.

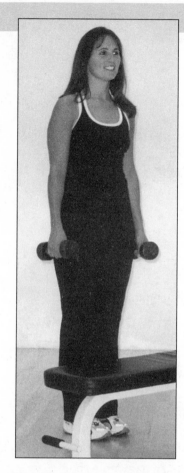

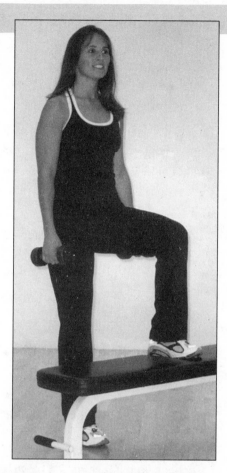

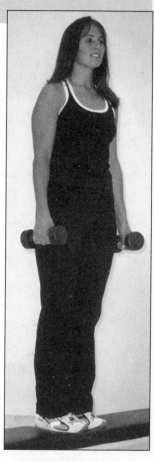

Dumbbell Step-Up—Start & Finish

Dumbbell Step-Up—Mid-Position One

Dumbbell Step-Up—Mid-Position Two

Band Hip Adduction

muscles	Inner thighs (hip adductors)
starting position	Sit on floor with band attached from secure anchor at right to right ankle with legs spread comfortably apart.
movement	Bring thighs together against resistance.
ending position	Right leg should be as close to left leg as comfortable.
key points	■ Place hands on floor behind hips and keep midsection tensed for greater stability. ■ Keep exercise leg relatively straight throughout exercise. ■ Exhale as you bring your thigh toward your body in two seconds, and inhale as you move your thigh away from your body in four seconds. ■ Perform repetitions with left leg after performing repetitions with right leg.

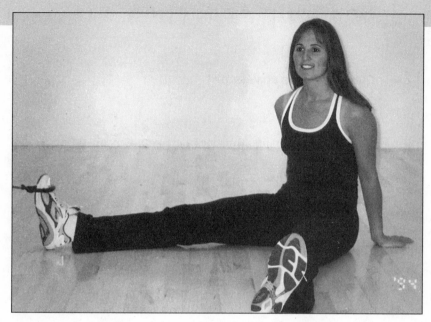

**Band Hip Adduction—
Start**

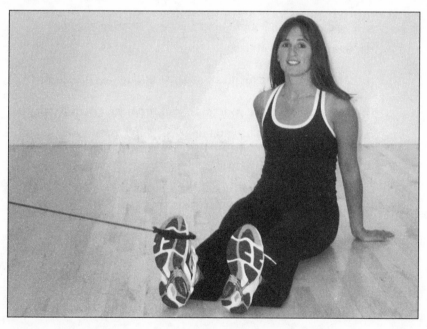

**Band Hip Adduction—
Finish**

Band Hip Abduction

muscles	Outer thighs (hip abductors)
starting position	Sit on floor with band attached from secure anchor at left to right ankle with legs together.
movement	Spread thighs apart against resistance.
ending position	Right leg should be as far from left leg as comfortable.
key points	▪ Place hands on floor behind hips, and keep midsection tensed for greater stability.
	▪ Keep exercise leg relatively straight throughout exercise.
	▪ Exhale as you move your thigh away from your body in two seconds, and inhale as you bring your thigh toward your body in four seconds.
	▪ Perform repetitions with left leg after performing repetitions with right leg.

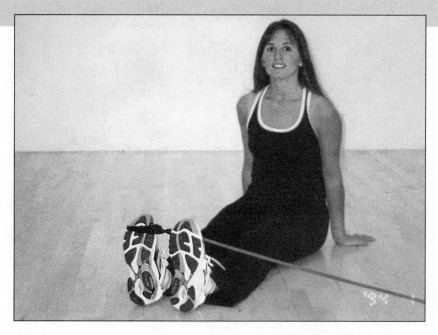

**Band Hip Abduction—
Start**

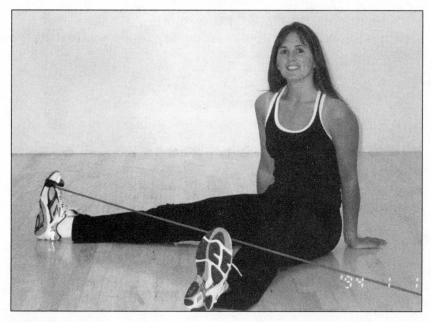

**Band Hip Abduction—
Finish**

Dumbbell Bench Press

muscles

Chest (pectoralis major)

Shoulders (anterior deltoid)

Rear arms (triceps)

starting position

Lie face-up on bench with feet on floor or step and dumbbells in hands just above broadest area of chest and about shoulder width apart.

movement

Push hands upward from chest level until arms are extended above chest.

ending position

Arms should be fully extended above broadest area of chest.

key points

- Keep hips and head on bench at all times.

- Keep wrists firm and in line with forearms throughout exercise.

- Keep elbows away from sides throughout exercise.

- Exhale as you lift the dumbbells in two seconds, and inhale as you lower the dumbbells in four seconds.

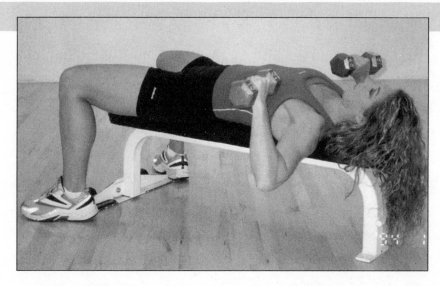

Dumbbell Bench
Press—Start

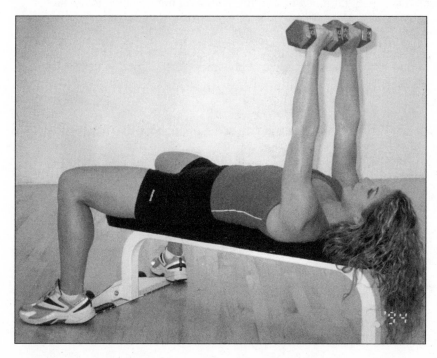

Dumbbell Bench
Press—Finish

Dumbbell Bent Row

muscles

Upper back (latissimus dorsi, rhomboids, middle trapezius)
Shoulders (posterior deltoid)
Front arm (biceps)

starting position

Place left hand and left knee on bench so that back is parallel to floor, and hold dumbbell with extended right arm directly below shoulder.

movement

Pull dumbbell upward from straight-arm position to chest.

ending position

Dumbbell should be at chest level with right arm flexed.

key points

- Keep head in line with spine throughout exercise.

- Keep wrists firm and in line with forearms throughout exercise.

- Keep elbows away from sides throughout exercise.

- Exhale as you lift the dumbbell in two seconds, and inhale as you lower the dumbbell in four seconds.

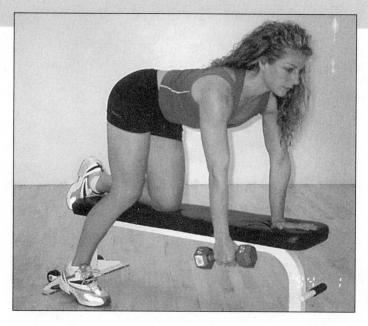

Dumbbell Bent Row—Start

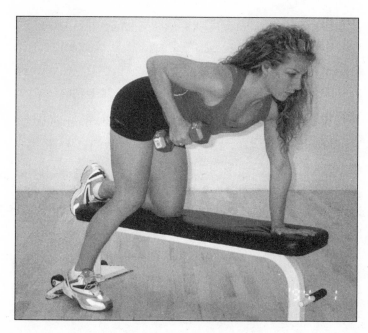

Dumbbell Bent Row—Finish

Dumbbell Overhead Press

muscles

Shoulders (deltoids)

Rear arm (triceps)

Neck (upper trapezius)

starting position

Stand with feet about shoulder width apart, holding dumbbells just above shoulders.

movement

Push dumbbells upward from just above shoulder level until arms are extended above shoulders.

ending position

Arms should be extended above shoulders.

key points

- Do not arch your back during the lifting action.

- Keep wrists firm and in line with forearms throughout exercise.

- Exhale as you lift the dumbbells in two seconds, and inhale as you lower the dumbbells in four seconds.

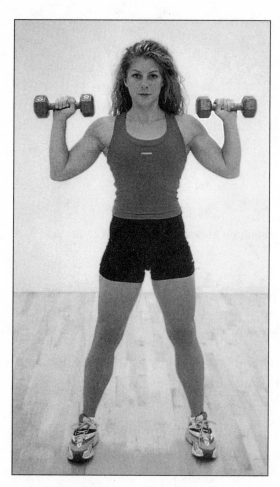

Dumbbell Overhead Press—Start

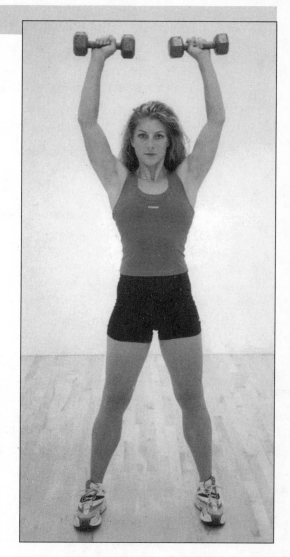

Dumbbell Overhead Press—Finish

Body Weight Trunk Extension

muscles

Lower back (erector spinae)

starting position

Lie face-down on floor with hands clasped loosely beneath chin.

movement

Move torso upward from front-lying position to trunk extended position.

ending position

Torso should be extended upward as far as comfortable.

key points

- Keep head in line with spine throughout exercise.

- Use arms to assist in torso lifting movements if necessary.

- Exhale as you lift your torso in two seconds, and inhale as you lower your torso in four seconds.

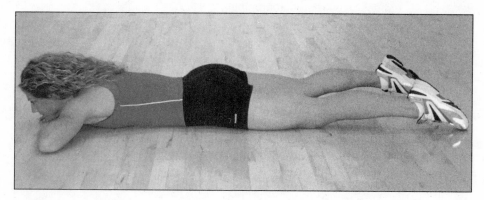

Body Weight Trunk Extension—Start

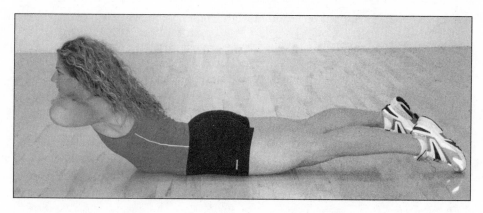

Body Weight Trunk Extension—Finish

Body Weight Trunk Curl

muscles	Midsection (rectus abdominis)
starting position	Lie face-up on floor with hands clasped loosely behind head, knees bent up to 90 degrees, and feet hip width apart.
movement	Move torso upward from back-lying position to trunk flexed position.
ending position	Torso should be flexed upward as far as comfortable.
key points	▪ Keep head in line with torso throughout exercise. ▪ Press lower back into floor as you curl shoulders off the floor. ▪ Exhale as you lift your torso in two seconds, and inhale as you lower your torso in four seconds.

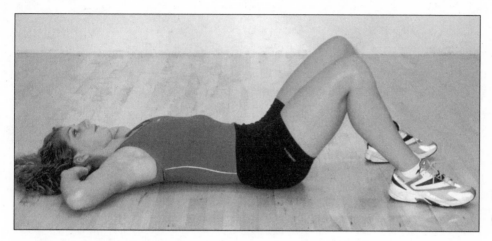

**Body Weight Trunk
Curl—Start**

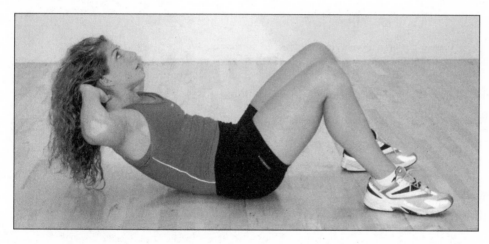

**Body Weight Trunk
Curl—Finish**

7 | Stretching Your Benefits

WE recently discovered that adding stretching exercise to the strength training program produces double benefits. We were aware that stretching exercise is the best way to increase joint flexibility, which is an important component of overall physical fitness. As you would expect, our research subjects who stretched after each strength exercise increased their joint flexibility more than the subjects who did not stretch.

However, we were surprised to learn that the research subjects who performed both strength training and stretching exercises also increased their muscle strength more than the subjects who did only strength training. In three separate studies with a total of 155 participants, those who stretched experienced almost 20 percent greater strength gains than those who did not stretch.

In addition to greater improvements in muscle strength and joint flexibility, the subjects who stretched between exercises reported enhanced workout enjoyment, as they found the stretching exercises relaxing.

The basic concept of the stretching component is to perform a 20-second static stretch for the muscles just worked before moving to the next exercise station. Because most people take about a minute rest between successive strength exercises, the 20-second stretches fit neatly into the workout program without adding more time to your training session. Also, all the stretches are designed to be done on or at the machines, which further facilitates training efficiency and convenience.

Performing the Stretching Exercises

Generally speaking, stretching tends to be reserved for either the beginning or end of an exercise session, usually following a thorough warm-up or after completing a comprehensive workout. Due to time constraints of a typical workout session (60 minutes), it is not uncommon for the stretching component to be seriously reduced or skipped entirely. This is unfortunate, because stretching has many benefits such as improving joint flexibility, reducing injury risk, relieving muscle tension, and enhancing strength gains. Our time-saving approach places your stretches between your strength exercises. You immediately perform a 20-second static stretch for the muscle group just trained on the Nautilus machine. For example, you follow the Leg Extension exercise with a stretch for the quadriceps muscles, and you follow the Leg Curl exercise with a stretch for the hamstrings muscles.

Warm-Up
You may engage in a traditional warm-up, such as walking on a treadmill or cycling on a stationary bike for several minutes before you strength train and stretch. However, as long as you work the target muscles with strength exercise and

perform the stretches correctly, you can stretch with little fear of injury. The strength exercise warms up your target muscle group and actually prepares you for the upcoming stretch.

> **RECOMMENDATION:** Warm up target muscles by performing a specific strength exercise prior to your stretch.

Frequency

How often should you stretch? According to the American College of Sports Medicine, an effective stretching program requires two to three sessions per week. You will perform the at-machine stretching exercises three days per week, which should produce excellent results.

> **RECOMMENDATION:** Perform at-machine stretching three days per week as part of your overall exercise program.

Stretch Type

We prefer static stretching exercises because they are very safe, effective, and time-efficient. Simply stretch your muscles to the pain-free "end point" of movement and sustain each stretch for 20 seconds. Our recommended stretching exercises are described and illustrated in Chapter Nine. Remember to gently move into your stretched position and hold this posture for 20 seconds while the muscles relax and adapt to their new length.

> **RECOMMENDATION:** Perform 20-second static stretches after each strength exercise.

Sets

The single-set approach for the strength exercises applies to the stretching protocol as well. You simply complete one complementary stretch for each strength exercise. Like the strength workout, the added stretch component is both time-efficient and productive. The distributed stretches add less than 5 minutes to the total workout time. If you wish to spend more time stretching for greater flexibility, at the end of the 20 seconds, gently reach another half-inch and hold that position for an additional 10 seconds.

> **RECOMMENDATION:** Perform one static stretch for each strength exercise. Blending these modes of exercise is both productive and time-efficient.

Posture

Correct posture involves keeping your body in proper alignment while you train. Otherwise, any stretching or strengthening exercise can be more harmful than beneficial. By now you already know that fast exercise movements are less safe and less effective than controlled exercise actions. You should always feel both the strength and stretching exercises in your muscles rather than in your joints. Proper posture is essential for maintaining desirable body alignment while you perform your exercises. Key posture pointers are to keep your torso erect; sit with your ankles, knees, and hips at right angles; keep your head up; and keep your neck in a neutral position. You will find that correct posture facilitates proper performance of the strength and stretching exercises.

> **RECOMMENDATION:** Utilize good posture and correct body alignment to perform each stretch in proper form.

Movement Speed

You should perform the at-machine stretching exercises in the same slow, controlled manner as you do your Nautilus exercises. Avoiding momentum will allow your muscles to safely relax and stretch, whereas fast or bouncing movements will actually tighten your muscles and may cause unnecessary trauma to your muscles and joints.

Range of Motion

To gain greater flexibility, you must stretch through a full range of joint movement, as long as you do not push to the point of pain. The sensation is often described as a slight pull, a feeling of mild tension, or tautness. At this point, you will hold your stretch for 20 seconds. You should feel your muscles relax as the tension eases. If you sense the slightest discomfort, slowly release into a more comfortable position. Remember, stretching should never be painful. It should always feel good when performed properly.

Breathing Technique

Chapter Five presented the procedures for proper breathing while performing strength exercise. You should never hold your breath while lifting weights or even when you stretch. We recommend that you breathe normally throughout every stretching exercise.

Muscle Balance

What muscles should you stretch? In our cellulite reduction program, you will stretch the very same muscles you are strengthening. It's just as important to stretch all the major muscle groups in a balanced manner as it is to strengthen them. Training this way will create balance and symmetry within the human structure, which in turn prevents muscle imbalances that could lead to injury.

> **RECOMMENDATION:** Stretch all major muscle groups, namely the same muscles you are strengthening.

The Fight Against Cellulite

Strength training will build muscle, provide a firm foundation for the overlying fat, and increase your fat-burning potential. Based on our research, adding stretching to your strength workout increases your joint flexibility and enhances your strength development. As you will see, all aspects of the program work together in a synergistic manner that helps you attain better overall results.

The At-Machine Stretching Guidelines

one | **RECOMMENDATION:**

WARM-UP: Perform a strength exercise before each stretch exercise to warm up muscles.

Note: Avoid stretching cold muscles.

two | **RECOMMENDATION:**

FREQUENCY: Perform at-machine stretching three days per week on the same days you strength train.

Note: Make stretching an essential component of your regular exercise schedule.

three | RECOMMENDATION:

STRETCH TYPE: Perform simple static stretches that you hold for about 20 seconds.

Note: Avoid complex stretching maneuvers.

four | RECOMMENDATION:

SETS: Perform one stretch per strength exercise for a productive and timely workout.

Note: Avoid overstretching your muscles, tendons, and connective tissues.

five | RECOMMENDATION:

POSTURE: Emphasize good posture and proper body alignment with each stretch.

Note: Position yourself properly before beginning your stretch.

six | RECOMMENDATION:

MOVEMENT SPEED: Perform each stretch in a slow and controlled manner.

Note: Avoid bouncing and ballistic stretches.

seven | RECOMMENDATION:

RANGE OF MOTION: Perform each stretch through a full range of pain-free joint movement.

Note: Stretch only to the point of muscle relaxation, not to the point of discomfort.

eight   **RECOMMENDATION:**

BREATHING TECHNIQUE: Breathe normally throughout your stretching routine.

Note: Avoid holding your breath when stretching.

nine   **RECOMMENDATION:**

MUSCLE BALANCE: Stretch all major muscle groups of the upper and lower body.

Note: Stretch each muscle group that you strength train.

The Stretching Exercises

Stretching is an activity you can do any time—morning, noon, or night. However, many people avoid stretching because they simply don't have time for a lengthy flexibility workout. The good news is that stretching can be integrated into a strength workout whether you use machines, free weights, rubber bands, and tubing or perform body weight exercises at home. By stretching the muscles after each strength exercise, you experience overall body flexibility without adding any/much time to your training session. With this approach, you will be less likely to overlook this essential fitness component. Combining stretching and strength exercises is effective, efficient, and fun to do. Other advantages of doing static stretches between strength exercises include greater ease of movement due to increased flexibility and greater functional strength due to enhanced muscle-building stimulus.

The strength training exercises in Chapter Six each have specific stretches that are performed on or at the machine. These stretches are designed to stretch your hips, thighs, upper body, and midsection.

To help you perform these exercises safely and correctly, this section provides easy-to-follow instructions and illustrations of all the stretches. After you complete each strength exercise, stretch the same muscle using good form and technique. Hold the stretch for 20 seconds. Do not bounce. Stretch to a point of "mild" tension. The stretch should feel good, *not* painful. Relax into the stretch. Go only as far as you feel comfortable. Be sure to breathe normally throughout the stretch. Do not hold your breath while stretching.

Machine Stretches

Quadriceps Stretch

muscles

Front thigh (quadriceps)

starting position

Stand facing away from leg movement pad.

movement

Hook foot over leg movement pad or seat. Repeat stretch with opposite leg.

ending position

Hips should be moved forward with toes, knees, and hips facing front and knees aligned with supporting leg.

key points

- Hold on to machine for support.

- Lean forward slightly, carefully hooking foot over pad or seat to avoid cramping rear thigh muscles.

- Align head, neck, shoulders, as well as hips, knees, and ankles.

- Breathe as you press your hips forward.

- Hold stretch for 20 seconds.

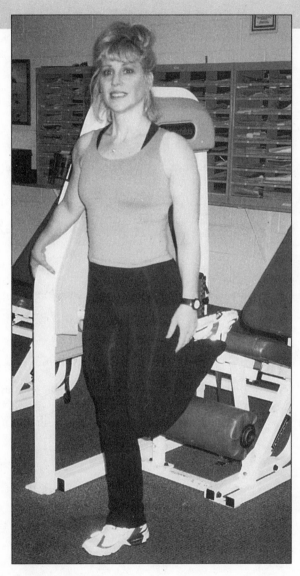

Quadriceps Stretch

Hamstrings Stretch

muscles	Rear thighs (hamstrings)
starting position	Remain seated, with arms resting on your thighs and legs extended and clamped between shin and ankle pads.
movement	Bend forward and reach for front thighs, roller, ankles, or toes.
ending position	Chest should be lifted, hips flexed forward, and toes pointed up.
key points	• Keep ankles at right angles throughout the stretch. • Do not round your back during the stretch. • Exhale as you bend forward. You should reach as far as you can go comfortably. • Hold stretch for 20 seconds.

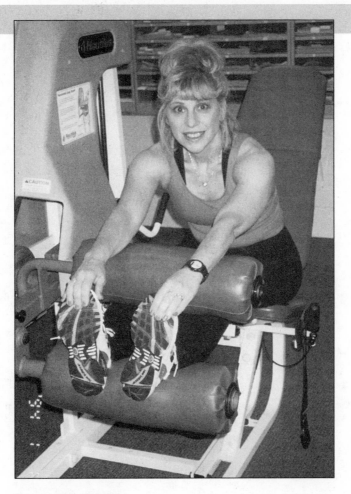

Hamstrings Stretch

Adductors Stretch

muscles

Inner thighs (hip adductors)

starting position

Remain seated with back against seatback, hands and legs outside movement pads, legs spread comfortably apart.

movement

Bend upper torso forward at hips.

ending position

Torso should be lifted, hips flexed forward, and legs spread comfortably apart.

key points

- After completing the strength exercise, adjust leg movement pad setting $1/2$–1 inch to lessen tension of inner thigh muscles.

- Exhale as you ease into your stretch.

- Hold stretch for 20 seconds.

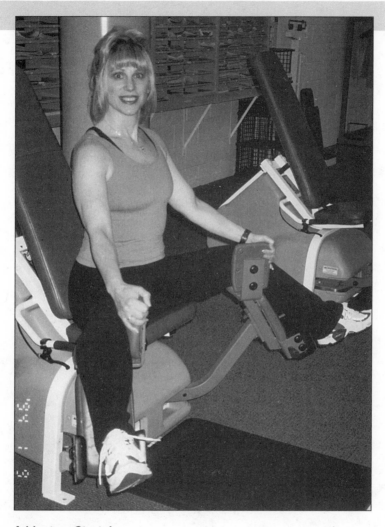

Adductors Stretch

Abductors Stretch

muscles

Outer thighs (hip abductors)

starting position

Remain seated with back against seatback, arms by your sides, legs resting on leg movement pads.

movement

Sit upright and cross right leg over outside of left knee (left leg is straight). Gently pull bent leg toward your left shoulder. Repeat stretch on opposite side.

ending position

Chest should be lifted and hips pressing down while bent leg is held fairly close to chest. Straight leg remains relaxed inside leg movement pad.

key points

- Use your arms to guide your bent leg toward your shoulder.

- Exhale as you ease into your stretch.

- Hold stretch for 20 seconds.

- Remember to stretch on both sides.

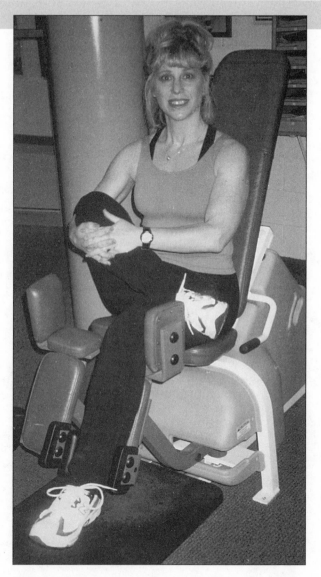

Abductors Stretch

Hip Stretch

muscles

Front thighs (quadriceps)
Rear thighs (hamstrings)
Buttocks (gluteals)

starting position

Remain seated with back against seatback. Place legs in relaxed butterfly position, hands positioned outside of legs.

movement

At bottom of foot plate, bring soles of feet together and let knees naturally fall open. Use hands to gently press thighs down.

ending position

Sit in butterfly position with hands pressing thighs downward.

key points

- Exhale and relax into your stretch.

- Hold stretch for 20 seconds.

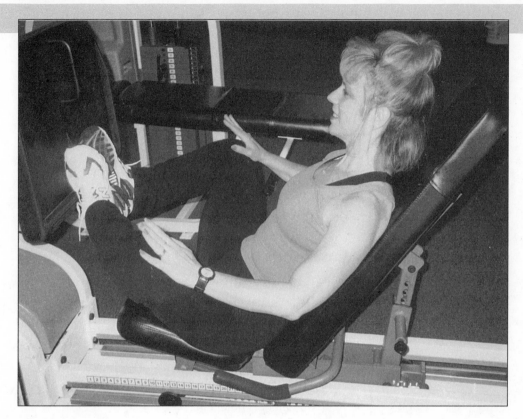

Hip Stretch

Chest Stretch

muscles	Chest (pectoralis major)
	Shoulders (anterior deltoid)
	Rear arms (triceps)
starting position	Sit upright on bench, feet on floor or step, arms by sides.
movement	Reach arms behind you to grasp handle bars.
ending position	Chest should be lifted, and arms should be fully extended behind your back.
key points	▪ Keep abdominals pulled in.
	▪ Maintain straight torso position. Do not arch low back.
	▪ Inhale as you push the chest out.
	▪ Hold stretch for 20 seconds.

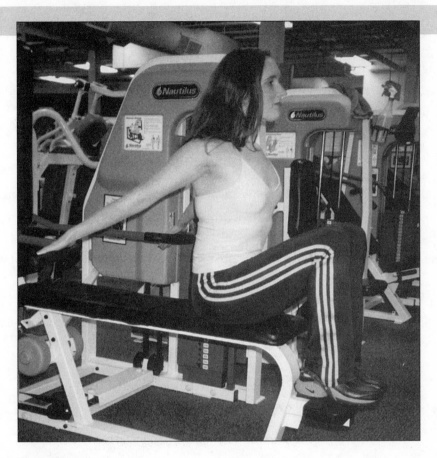

Chest Stretch

Upper Back Stretch

muscles

Upper back (latissimus dorsi, rhomboids, middle trapezius)

Shoulders (posterior deltoid)

Front arm (biceps)

starting position

Stand behind seat facing chest pad, arms slightly bent.

movement

Firmly grasp top of chest pad. Bend knees, and squat backward.

ending position

Arms should be fully extended, hips tucked, and mid-upper back rounded.

key points

- Legs should be hip width apart.

- Lead with your hips as you begin the stretch.

- Keep knees bent and in line with your ankle joints.

- Exhale while you tighten abdominals.

- Hold stretch for 20 seconds.

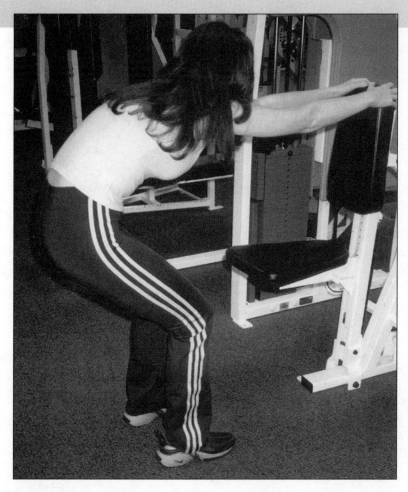

Upper Back Stretch

Shoulder Stretch

muscles

Shoulders (deltoids)

Rear arm (triceps)

Neck (upper trapezius)

starting position

Stand erect, feet staggered, facing away from handle bars.

movement

Stand erect, right leg bent in front, left leg in back, heel pressed against floor. Reach arms behind body to grasp lower handles.

ending position

Your right leg should be in front, your left leg in back (front knee bent, back leg straight), arms fully extended behind you, and chest lifted as you hold on to the handle bars.

key points

- Place right hand on right bar, left hand on left bar.

- Keep abdominals pulled in.

- Exhale as you push your chest out.

- Hold stretch for 20 seconds.

- You may place your left leg in front if you prefer this stance.

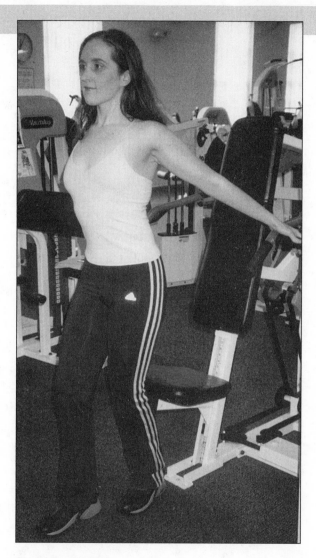

Shoulder Stretch

Low Back Stretch

muscles

Lower back (erector spinae)

starting position

Release seatback, and sit upright with hips against seatback and feet firmly planted.

movement

Hold on to edge of seat with both feet on foot plate or floor. Gently lower torso onto thighs.

ending position

Torso should be hanging down and resting on thighs, and hands should be reaching toward feet.

key points

- Allow head, neck, and shoulder muscles to relax.

- Round back.

- Exhale as you flex trunk forward.

- Hold stretch for 20 seconds.

- Rise from stretch slowly.

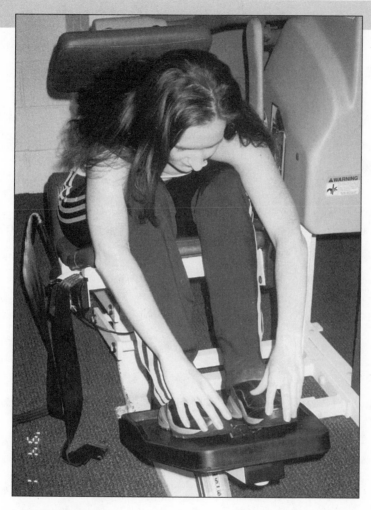

Low Back Stretch

Abdominal Stretch

muscles	Midsection (rectus abdominis)
starting position	Remain seated in an upright position, both arms resting on your thighs, palms facing down.
movement	Sit upright, place one hand over the other, and lift both arms over head.
ending position	Sit at edge of seat in erect position, hands clasped and arms stretched overhead.
key points	▪ Maintain natural curve of your spine during this stretch.
	▪ Relax your abdominal muscles.
	▪ Align fully extended arms next to your ears.
	▪ Exhale as you stretch.
	▪ Hold stretch for 20 seconds.

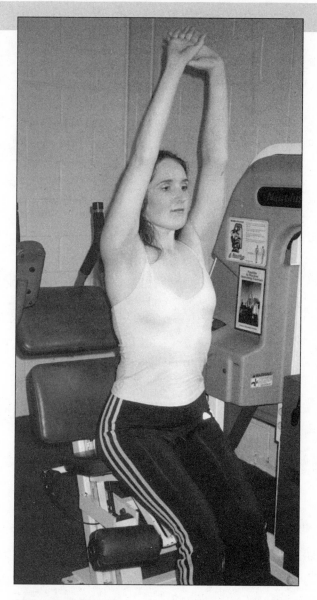

Abdominal Stretch

Free-Weight Stretches

Front Thigh Stretch

muscles	Front thigh (quadriceps)
starting position	Face away from bench or chair.
movement	Hook foot over bench or kitchen chair seat. Reverse positions.
ending position	Hips should be moved forward with toes, knees, and hips facing front and knees aligned with supporting leg.
key points	• Lean forward slightly, carefully hooking foot over bench or chair to avoid cramping rear thigh muscles. • Align head, neck, shoulders as well as hips, knees, and ankles. • Breathe as you press your hips forward. • Hold stretch for 20 seconds. • Stretch both legs.

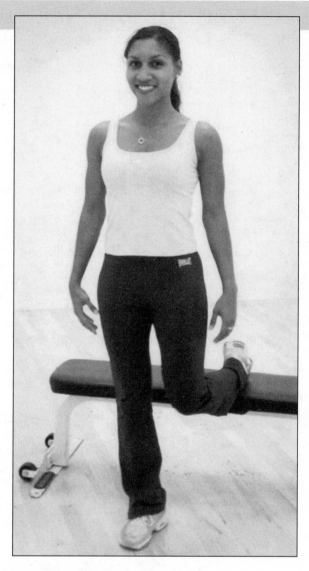

Front Thigh Stretch

Front Hip Stretch

muscles	Hip (iliopsoas) Rear thigh (hamstrings) Groin (inner thighs)
starting position	Stand facing bench or chair, and hold for support.
movement	Standing with one leg in front and the other in back, kneel on floor with back knee. Reverse positions.
ending position	In kneeling position, straighten arms on bench or chair as you press hips downward.
key points	• Keep your upper body erect while you straighten your arms and stretch your hip. • Breathe as you lower the front of your hips. • Hold stretch for 20 seconds. • Stretch both legs.

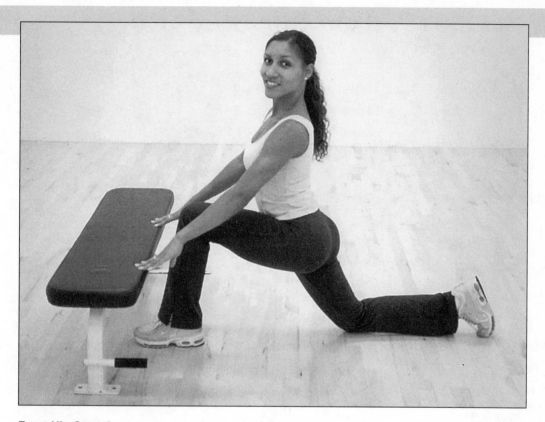

Front Hip Stretch

Lower Body Stretch

muscles
Rear thighs (hamstrings)
Buttocks (gluteals)
Lower back (erector spinae)

starting position
Lie on your back with both legs straight.

movement
Clasp your hands and hold back of bent thigh while straightening the opposite leg. Reverse positions.

ending position
Bent thigh should be pulled toward chest while opposite leg is outstretched and relaxed.

key points
- Keep your abdominals taut while you press your lower back against the floor.
- Relax your neck and shoulders.
- Hold this stretch for 20 seconds.
- Stretch both legs.

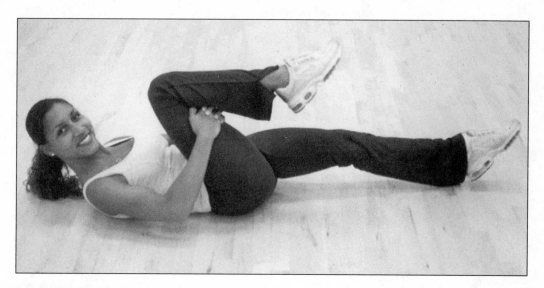

Lower Body Stretch

Groin Stretch

muscles

Inner thighs (hip adductors)

Lower back (erector spinae)

starting position

Sit on floor with soles of your feet together.

movement

Spread thighs apart.

ending position

With your back straight, hold onto your ankles, bend forward, and gently press your elbows down on the inside of your thighs.

key points

- With your elbows, push gently on your inner thighs rather than on your knees.

- Contract your abdominals as you exhale and lean forward.

- Relax and hold stretch for 20 seconds.

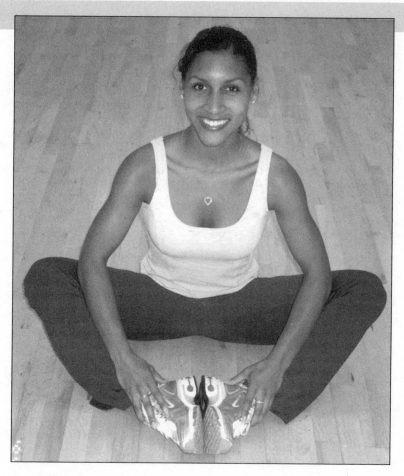

Groin Stretch

Outer Hip Stretch

muscles

Outer thigh (hip abductors)

starting position

Sit on floor with one leg straight and the other leg bent and resting on the outside of the opposite knee. Reverse positions.

movement

Cross one leg over the other.

ending position

With your back straight, hug your bent thigh and gently draw your knee across your chest toward your opposite shoulder.

key points

- At the same time you pull your knee across your body, exhale and press your hips down to feel the stretch along the side of your hip.

- Hold stretch for 20 seconds.

- Stretch both legs.

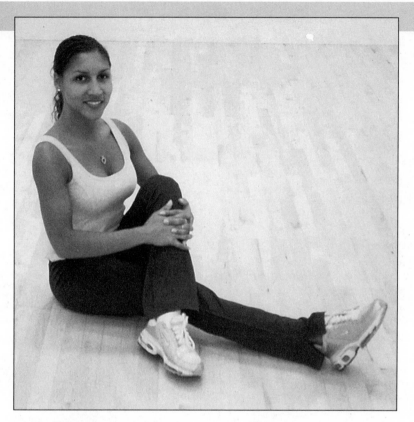

Outer Hip Stretch

Chest Stretch

muscles

Chest (pectoralis major)

Shoulders (anterior deltoid)

Arms (biceps, forearms)

starting position

Lie face-up on bench or cushions with feet on floor and arms resting by your sides.

movement

Outstretch arms.

ending position

Arms outstretched, palms facing the ceiling, with chest up and shoulder blades together.

key points

- Keep hips and head on bench at all times.

- Inhale as your chest expands.

- Relax your arms, and let gravity gently pull your arms downward.

- Breathe and hold stretch for 20 seconds.

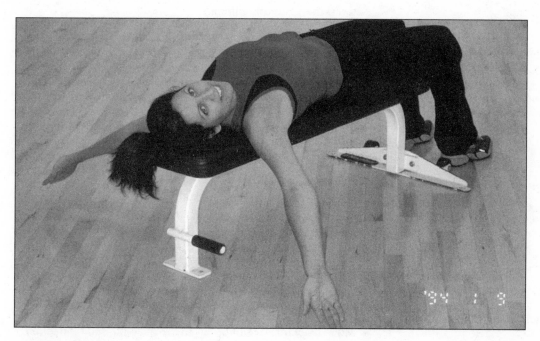

Chest Stretch

Upper Back Stretch

muscles
Upper back (latissimus dorsi, rhomboids, middle trapezius)
Shoulders (posterior deltoids)
Front arm (biceps)

starting position
Kneel about six inches away from bench or chair with both hands holding far edge of bench or seat.

movement
Pull back as you reach arms forward.

ending position
Firmly holding onto the bench, slowly sit back onto your heels as you straighten both arms.

key points
- Move body (hips) right or left to increase stretch on desired side.

- Relax feet.

- Exhale, and draw in your abdominals as you ease into the stretch.

- Hold stretch for 20 seconds.

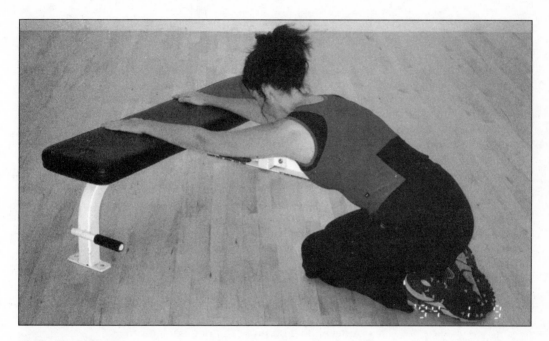

Upper Back Stretch

Shoulder Stretch

muscles

Shoulders (deltoids)

Arms (biceps)

Chest (pectoralis major)

starting position

Sit upright on bench or chair with feet firmly planted and arms resting by your sides.

movement

Straighten arms behind your back and lift chest.

ending position

Grasp bench with right hand on right edge and left hand on left edge, several inches behind hips.

key points

- Arms should be fully extended behind you.

- Pull abdominals in as you expand your chest.

- Slide arms backward until you feel the stretch in the arms and shoulders.

- Exhale and hold stretch for 20 seconds.

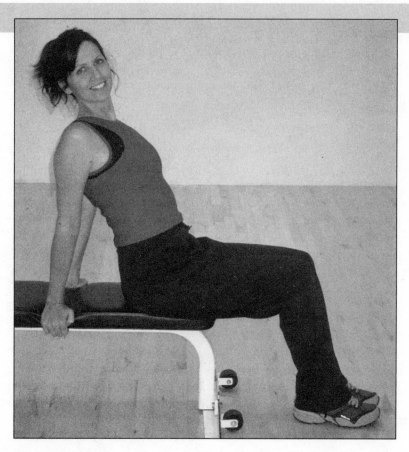

Shoulder Stretch

Lower Back Stretch

muscles	Lower back (erector spinae)
starting position	Lie face-up on floor with both knees bent, feet hip width apart about six inches away from your hips, with toes and knees facing front.
movement	Bring bent knees up toward chest.
ending position	Hold back of thighs as you gently pull your knees in toward your chest.
key points	■ Draw abdominals in as you exhale. ■ Press hips down as you bring knees toward chest. ■ Hold stretch for 20 seconds.

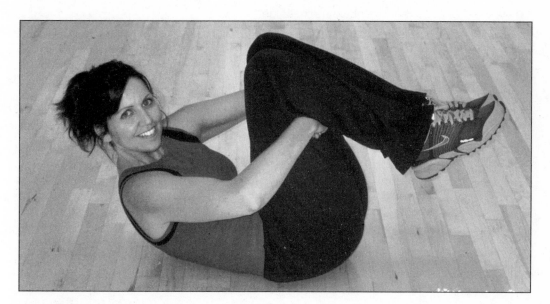

Lower Back Stretch

Abdominal Stretch

muscles
Abdominals (rectus abdominis)
Shoulders (deltoids)
Arms (biceps, forearms)

starting position
Lie face-up on floor with knees bent and arms resting by your sides.

movement
Extend arms and legs.

ending position
Extend arms overhead and straighten legs, making yourself as long as possible.

key points
- Exhale and pull your abdominals in as you stretch.
- Relax your neck and shoulders as you reach overhead.
- Hold stretch for 20 seconds.

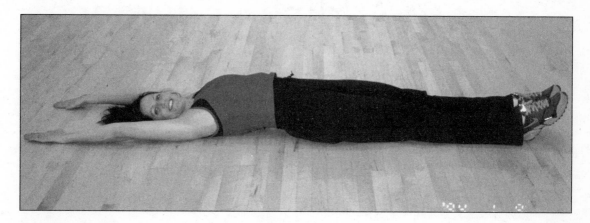

Abdominal Stretch

8 | Adding Endurance Exercise

LIKE strength training, endurance exercise is another essential component of your cellulite reduction program. As you are aware, strength training builds muscle, recharges metabolism, and enables you to burn more calories during your workout, after your workout, and all day long. Although endurance training has little effect on your resting metabolic rate, it definitely enhances energy use during your exercise session. Endurance exercise also provides cardiovascular conditioning, which is an important health benefit.

Endurance training, also known as aerobic activity, includes walking, jogging, cycling, stepping, rowing, and similar forms of large-muscle, continuous-movement exercise. Twenty minutes of jogging burns approximately 220 calories, compared to about 200 calories for 25 minutes of circuit strength training. A combined 45-minute training session (25 minutes of strength exercise plus 20 minutes of endurance exercise) may, therefore, use more than 400 calories.

Strength exercise for the muscular system and endurance exercise for the cardiovascular system are highly complementary activities. Although both require physical effort, strength training emphasizes the anaerobic energy system and endurance training emphasizes the aerobic energy system. The anaerobic energy system (without oxygen) enables you to perform high-effort exercise, such as strength training, for relatively short periods of time (90 seconds or less). The aerobic energy system (with oxygen) enables you to perform low- to moderate-effort exercise, such as walking and jogging, for relatively long periods of time (several minutes to several hours). Our research has revealed almost identical results regardless of the activity order. In other words, whether you do strength exercise followed by endurance exercise or endurance exercise followed by strength exercise is largely a matter of personal preference.

Like strength training, there are key principles for performing endurance exercise in a safe and productive manner. The following recommendations should minimize the risks and maximize the benefits of your endurance training program.

Principle of Progression: Duration

Obviously, the words *endurance* and *duration* are closely related. Endurance training typically refers to moderate effort aerobic activities that can be continued for 20 minutes or longer. Exercising in this manner is beneficial for calorie burning and cardiovascular conditioning. However, not everyone is capable of a 20-minute endurance exercise session. We recommend beginning with as little aerobic activity as you can comfortably perform while carrying on a normal conversation. Whether this is 2 minutes or 10 minutes makes no difference, because you will gradually progress to longer exercise sessions.

The progression principle may be applied in one- to two-minute increments on a week-by-week basis. For example, if you perform six minutes of stationary cycling your first week of training, you may increase to eight minutes your second week of training, and to 10 minutes your third week of training. Adding two more minutes each week will bring you to 20 minutes of endurance exercise by your second month of training.

> RECOMMENDATION: Gradually increase the duration of your endurance exercise sessions by one to two minutes per week, until you can complete 20 minutes of continuous aerobic activity.

Principle of Progression: Intensity

Increasing the exercise duration is the first step in developing your cardiovascular fitness. However, many people extend their exercise duration too far or too quickly and encounter difficulty maintaining their training motivation. We prefer a moderate exercise duration (20 to 30 minutes of continuous aerobic activity), with gradual increases in the exercise intensity. Enhancing your endurance exercise is not as difficult as it appears, because most people naturally pick up their pace as they become better conditioned.

For example, you may begin a treadmill-walking program at a two-mile-per-hour pace. However, after a couple weeks of training, this pace will probably feel too slow, and you will set the speed for 2.5 miles per hour. After another two weeks of training, you may increase the pace to three miles per hour. The faster pace provides higher-intensity training that burns more calories and enhances cardiovascular fitness.

Consider that a two-mile-per-hour walking pace burns about 200 calories over an hour training session. However, a four-mile-per-hour walking pace burns more than 200 calories in just a half-hour training session. Training at a faster pace certainly makes sense for time-pressured people, as you can use more calories in shorter workouts.

One way to gauge your rate of intensity progression is known as the talk test. When you can talk normally as you exercise, you are ready to make a small increase in the training intensity. If you can talk in short sentences but not in continuous conversation, the exercise intensity is high enough. If you have difficulty blurting out brief phrases, you should reduce your training intensity to a less-demanding effort level.

A more precise means for evaluating your exercise intensity is heart rate monitoring. This can be easily accomplished by wearing a heart rate monitoring device, or by simply taking your pulse during the exercise session. Your recommended exercise heart rate is between 70 and 80 percent of your maximum heart rate. Because your maximum heart rate decreases about one beat per year as you age, different people have different ranges for exercise heart rates. As shown in Table 8.1, the exercise heart rate range for a 40-year-old-woman is between 126 and 144 heart beats per minute, whereas the exercise heart rate range for a 60-year-old woman is 112 to 128 heart beats per minute. To calculate your personal

Table 8.1

Recommended exercise heart rate ranges for people between 20 and 80 years of age.

Age (years)	20	30	40	50	60	70	80
Maximum heart rate (beats/ minute)	200	190	180	170	160	150	140
Exercise heart rate range (beats/ minute)	140–160	134–152	126–144	119–136	112–128	105–120	98–112

exercise heart rate range more precisely, subtract your age (years) from 220 and multiply this number by 0.7 and 0.8 (70 to 80 percent).

Generally speaking, you should set your exercise intensity so that your heart rate is in the middle of your training range. As you become better conditioned, this exercise intensity will be less demanding and will elicit lower training heart rates. When your exercise heart rate drops below your training range, it is time to make a modest increase in your exercise intensity.

For example, a 50-year-old woman training at level two on the stationary cycle has an exercise heart rate of 125 beats per minute, which is in the middle of her range (see Table 8.1). However, after three weeks of training, level two cycling elevates her heart rate to only 115 beats per minute. This is an indication that she should progress to level three on the stationary cycle. When her exercise heart rate again drops below 119 beats per minute, she should begin training at level four.

> RECOMMENDATION: Gradually increase the intensity of your endurance training program. Higher effort levels are indicated when you can talk normally while you exercise, or when your exercise heart rate falls below your age-related training range.

Principle of Progression: Exercise Selection

If you are overweight or out of shape, you may consider a progression in the type of exercise you perform, beginning with a less-demanding aerobic activity such as stationary cycling. Because the cycle supports your body weight, it is easier to perform than weight-bearing exercises such as treadmill walking or stair climbing. Stationary cycling involves only external resistance, and you can easily adjust your effort level from freewheeling to really hard pedal pushing.

The next piece of equipment in our suggested progression is the treadmill, set for slow walking on a level surface. While walking requires body weight control, the mostly horizontal movements should not be too demanding, and the weight-bearing activity is more beneficial for bone health. As you become more fit, you may gradually increase the treadmill elevation so you are walking up steeper inclines.

After mastering incline walking, you should be ready for a stair-climbing machine. Stair climbing requires you to lift your body weight vertically against gravity, which, like rope jumping, is a more challenging aerobic activity.

Once you can confidently perform these exercises, you may want to consider cross-training. That is, you may do stationary cycling on Mondays, treadmill walking on Wednesdays, and stair climbing on Fridays. Alternating aerobic activities reduces the risk of overtraining injuries and makes your exercise program more interesting.

RECOMMENDATION: Begin your endurance exercise program with a less-demanding activity such as stationary cycling and progress to more challenging activities such as treadmill walking and stair climbing.

Principle of Progression: Frequency

Because endurance exercise is less stressful to your muscles than strength exercise, you recover more quickly between training sessions. Unlike a strenuous strength workout that requires two days for muscle recovery and rebuilding, most people can perform moderate effort endurance exercise every day if they choose to do so. However, we do not recommend that you start with such frequent training sessions.

We prefer beginning with a three-day-per-week training schedule for both your strength exercise and aerobic activity. Given about 25 minutes to complete your strength workout and between 20 to 30 minutes of endurance exercise, your total training session should take between 45 to 55 minutes. Although this is not an unreasonable amount of activity time, you will probably appreciate a full recovery day between workouts.

Once you have established a consistent Monday-Wednesday-Friday or Tuesday-Thursday-Saturday exercise schedule, you may wish to add on an extra day or two of aerobic activity. If you do, consider alternating exercises on successive days. For example, if you are jogging on Monday, Wednesday, and Friday, we suggest cycling on the other days you choose to exercise. This reduces the risk of overusing specific muscle groups and enhances recovery between training sessions.

> RECOMMENDATION: Perform three endurance exercise sessions per week as standard training. If you choose to do more frequent aerobic activity, alternate exercises on successive days to prevent overtraining.

Principle of Warm-Up and Cool-Down

To make a smooth transition from your resting state to sustained aerobic activity, you should always precede your endurance exercise with a progressive warm-up. For most practical purposes, the recommended warm-up procedure begins with a few calisthenics exercises such as trunk curls for the midsection muscles and half-squats for the leg muscles. This may be followed by some gentle stretching and bending exercises to loosen up your major muscle groups and joint structures. The final phase of the warm-up involves a few minutes of your selected endurance exercise at a lower level of intensity. For example, if you plan to cycle for 15 minutes at level six (150 watts of power output/effort level), you may warm up for two minutes at level two (50 watts) and two minutes at level four (100 watts) before entering your training zone. Doing so prepares you physically and mentally for your workout and avoids abrupt physiological demands on your cardiovascular system.

When you are exercising, your heart is pumping blood to the working muscles at a much higher rate and you may be using oxygen at more than 10 times your resting level. In addition to the faster and stronger pumping action of your heart, previously closed capillaries are opened to accommodate greater blood flow. The continuous movement of your muscles also provides a pumping function, facilitating blood return to your heart by their squeezing action against your veins.

While this process is perfectly balanced during your workout, suddenly stopping your exercise session can have undesirable consequences. For example, when you stop pedaling the bike, your heart continues to pump large supplies of blood to the leg muscles. However, because you are no longer moving your legs, these muscles cannot assist in returning blood to your heart. As a result, blood accumulates in the legs and seriously diminishes blood flow to the rest of the body, including your head. The reduced blood circulation may produce feelings of light-headedness or nausea.

Fortunately, by performing a few minutes of cool-down activity, you can avoid these problems. The main purpose of the cool-down period is to keep your leg muscles moving with gradually decreasing intensity to maintain balanced blood circulation as your heart returns to resting function. Other objectives of the cool-down include systematic reduction in muscular activity followed by muscle relaxation to help you leave the workout feeling invigorated rather than fatigued.

The first phase of your cool-down should simply be an extension of your training exercise at a gradually decreasing exertion level. For example, if you have just cycled for 15 minutes at level six (150 watts), spend a minute at level five (125 watts), another minute at level four (100 watts), a minute at level three (75 watts), and another minute at level two (50 watts) before you stop pedaling.

We always recommend walking for a couple minutes as part of your cool-down, followed by a few gentle stretching exercises such as the Figure "4" Stretch and the Letter "T" Stretch (please see Appendix B). Generally speaking, your heart rate should be close to its resting level (typically 70 to 90 beats per minute) by the conclusion of your cool-down.

As a final note, always use good (upright) posture when performing endurance exercise. Slouching can definitely decrease your training benefits, making the exercise less effective and less enjoyable.

Summary of Endurance Exercise Guidelines

If you incorporate the following principles of endurance exercise, you should experience safe, effective, and enjoyable training sessions. Keep in mind that your aerobic activities should be performed at moderate effort levels.

one | RECOMMENDATION:

DURATION: Gradually increase the duration of your endurance exercise sessions by one to two minutes per week, until you can complete 20 minutes of continuous aerobic activity.

Note: Perform longer periods of endurance exercise if you desire, but don't overdo this component of your total training program.

two | RECOMMENDATION:

INTENSITY: Gradually increase the intensity of your endurance training program. Higher effort levels are indicated when you can talk normally while you exercise, or when your exercise heart rate falls below your age-related training range.

Note: Avoid training at uncomfortable levels of exercise intensity when doing aerobic activity.

three   **RECOMMENDATION:**

EXERCISE SELECTION: Begin your endurance exercise program with a less-demanding activity such as stationary cycling and progress to more challenging activities such as treadmill walking and stair climbing.

Note: Vary your endurance exercises to prevent boredom and reduce the risk of overuse injuries.

four   **RECOMMENDATION:**

FREQUENCY: Perform three endurance exercise sessions per week as standard training. If you choose to do more frequent aerobic activity, alternate exercises on successive days to prevent overtraining.

Note: Schedule at least one rest day each week to ensure sufficient recovery from endurance exercise activities.

five   **RECOMMENDATION:**

WARM-UP AND COOL-DOWN: Endurance exercise should be preceded by a few minutes of warm-up activity and followed by a few minutes of cool-down activity to facilitate smooth transitions between inactive and active physical states.

Note: Always take time to gradually warm up and cool down, even if you must reduce the higher-effort segment of your training session.

9 | The No More Cellulite Exercise Program

STRENGTH training, stretching exercise, and aerobic activity are the three key components of physical fitness. A strong and flexible muscular system coupled with a well-conditioned cardiovascular system should make you look better, feel better, and function better. In addition, there is ample evidence that a well-rounded fitness program can enhance both the quality and the quantity of your life.

We have discovered that a specifically designed fitness program featuring strength training, stretching exercise, and aerobic activity can significantly improve your cellulite situation. Our anti-cellulite program includes specific exercises for target areas, as well as for total body training. The specific strength exercises replace muscle where it has been lost, providing a firm foundation for an attractive figure. Along with the triple-reducing effect of strength training (calories burned during the workout, after the workout, and all day long), the endurance exercise increases your energy expenditure and expedites fat loss.

Although the essential aspect of an anti-cellulite program is effectiveness, it is also important to have time-efficient training sessions. Lengthy workouts typically become unmanageable in terms of scheduling factors, physical fatigue, and mental focus. We have, therefore, developed a successful cellulite reduction program that requires only 45 minutes for completion. If you train on a Monday-Wednesday-Friday schedule, you will spend just over two hours a week in exercise activity. This is a much better use of your time than thinking about dieting all day, every day.

This chapter presents our recommended exercise program for winning the cellulite battle. We realize that few people are fit enough to perform the whole training program initially. For this reason, we introduce the exercise components in a progressive sequence that allows your body to safely and successfully adapt to each workout. Depending on your personal fitness level, you may progress faster or slower than our suggested training schedule. You may also interchange the endurance exercises as you desire, based on your activity preference, fitness level, and equipment availability.

Recommended Exercise Program Using Weightstack Machines

Beginning with five specific exercises for your hips and thighs, we recommend making workout modifications every Monday of successive training weeks. Although we provide suggested weightloads for each strength exercise, be sure to adjust the resistance according to your present muscular ability. An appropriate weightload is one that you can perform 10 to 15 times in proper form. If you can do fewer than 10 repetitions, the resistance is too heavy; if you can do more than 15 repetitions, the resistance is too light. Generally, you should increase your training weightload by about 5 percent whenever you complete 15 good repetitions.

Week One MONDAY-WEDNESDAY-FRIDAY

STRENGTH

Exercise	Major Muscles	Training Protocol	Suggested Weightload
Leg Extension	Front thighs	1 set of 10 to 15 repetitions	35.0 lbs
Leg Curl	Rear thighs	1 set of 10 to 15 repetitions	35.0 lbs
Hip Adduction	Inner thighs	1 set of 10 to 15 repetitions	47.5 lbs
Hip Abduction	Outer thighs	1 set of 10 to 15 repetitions	37.5 lbs
Leg Press	Buttocks Front thighs Rear thighs	1 set of 10 to 15 repetitions	75.0 lbs

STRETCHING

Exercise	Major Muscles	Training Protocol
Quadriceps Stretch	Front thighs	10-second static stretch following Leg Extension exercise
Hamstrings Stretch	Rear thighs	10-second static stretch following Leg Curl exercise
Adductors Stretch	Inner thighs	10-second static stretch following Hip Adduction exercise
Abductors Stretch	Outer thighs	10-second static stretch following Hip Abduction exercise
Hip Stretch	Buttocks	10-second static stretch following Leg Press exercise

ENDURANCE

Exercise	Warm-Up Time	Training Time	Cool-Down Time
Stationary Cycling	3 to 5 minutes easy effort	6 to 10 minutes moderate effort	3 to 5 minutes easy effort

140   NO MORE CELLULITE

Week Two   MONDAY-WEDNESDAY-FRIDAY

Exercise	Major Muscles	Training Protocol	Suggested Weightload
Leg Extension	Front thighs	1 set of 10 to 15 repetitions	37.5 lbs
Leg Curl	Rear thighs	1 set of 10 to 15 repetitions	37.5 lbs
Hip Adduction	Inner thighs	1 set of 10 to 15 repetitions	50.0 lbs
Hip Abduction	Outer thighs	1 set of 10 to 15 repetitions	40.0 lbs
Leg Press	Buttocks Front thighs Rear thighs	1 set of 10 to 15 repetitions	80.0 lbs
Abdominal Curl	Midsection	1 set of 10 to 15 repetitions	37.5 lbs
Low Back Extension	Lower back	1 set of 10 to 15 repetitions	37.5 lbs

STRETCHING

Exercise	Major Muscles	Training Protocol
Quadriceps Stretch	Front thighs	10-second static stretch following Leg Extension exercise
Hamstrings Stretch	Rear thighs	10-second static stretch following Leg Curl exercise
Adductors Stretch	Inner thighs	10-second static stretch following Hip Adduction exercise
Abductors Stretch	Outer thighs	10-second static stretch following Hip Abduction exercise
Hip Stretch	Buttocks	10-second static stretch following Leg Press exercise
Abdominal Stretch	Midsection	10-second static stretch following Abdominal Curl exercise
Low Back Stretch	Lower back	10-second static stretch following Low Back Extension exercise

Exercise	Warm-Up Time	Training Time	Cool-Down Time
Stationary Cycling	3 to 5 minutes easy effort	8 to 12 minutes moderate effort	3 to 5 minutes easy effort

Week Three MONDAY-WEDNESDAY-FRIDAY

STRENGTH

Exercise	Major Muscles	Training Protocol	Suggested Weightload
Leg Extension	Front thighs	1 set of 10 to 15 repetitions	40.0 lbs
Leg Curl	Rear thighs	1 set of 10 to 15 repetitions	40.0 lbs
Hip Adduction	Inner thighs	1 set of 10 to 15 repetitions	52.5 lbs
Hip Abduction	Outer thighs	1 set of 10 to 15 repetitions	42.5 lbs
Leg Press	Buttocks Front thighs Rear thighs	1 set of 10 to 15 repetitions	85.0 lbs
Bench Press	Chest Shoulders Rear arms	1 set of 10 to 15 repetitions	32.5 lbs
Seated Row	Upper back Front arms	1 set of 10 to 15 repetitions	47.5 lbs
Overhead Press	Shoulders Rear arms	1 set of 10 to 15 repetitions	27.5 lbs
Abdominal Curl	Midsection	1 set of 10 to 15 repetitions	40.0 lbs
Low Back Extension	Lower back	1 set of 10 to 15 repetitions	40.0 lbs

Exercise	Major Muscles	Training Protocol
Quadriceps Stretch	Front thighs	15-second static stretch following Leg Extension exercise
Hamstrings Stretch	Rear thighs	15-second static stretch following Leg Curl exercise
Adductors Stretch	Inner thighs	15-second static stretch following Hip Adduction exercise
Abductors Stretch	Outer thighs	15-second static stretch following Hip Abduction exercise
Hip Stretch	Buttocks	15-second static stretch following Leg Press exercise
Chest Stretch	Front torso	15-second static stretch following Bench Press exercise
Upper Back Stretch	Rear torso	15-second static stretch following Seated Row exercise
Shoulder Stretch	Shoulders	15-second static stretch following Overhead Press exercise
Abdominal Stretch	Midsection	15-second static stretch following Abdominal Curl exercise
Low Back Stretch	Lower back	15-second static stretch following Low Back Extension exercise

ENDURANCE

Exercise	Warm-Up Time	Training Time	Cool-Down Time
Treadmill Walking	3 to 5 minutes easy effort	10 to 14 minutes moderate effort	3 to 5 minutes easy effort

Week Four   MONDAY-WEDNESDAY-FRIDAY

Exercise	Major Muscles	Training Protocol	Suggested Weightload
Leg Extension	Front thighs	1 set of 10 to 15 repetitions	42.5 lbs
Leg Curl	Rear thighs	1 set of 10 to 15 repetitions	42.5 lbs
Hip Adduction	Inner thighs	1 set of 10 to 15 repetitions	55.0 lbs
Hip Abduction	Outer thighs	1 set of 10 to 15 repetitions	45.0 lbs
Leg Press	Buttocks Front Thighs Rear thighs	1 set of 10 to 15 repetitions	90.0 lbs
Bench Press	Chest Shoulders Rear arms	1 set of 10 to 15 repetitions	35.0 lbs
Seated Row	Upper back Front arms	1 set of 10 to 15 repetitions	50.0 lbs
Overhead Press	Shoulders Rear arms	1 set of 10 to 15 repetitions	30.0 lbs
Abdominal Curl	Midsection	1 set of 10 to 15 repetitions	42.5 lbs
Low Back Extension	Lower back	1 set of 10 to 15 repetitions	42.5 lbs

STRETCHING

Exercise	Major Muscles	Training Protocol
Quadriceps Stretch	Front thighs	20-second static stretch following Leg Extension exercise
Hamstrings Stretch	Rear thighs	20-second static stretch following Leg Curl exercise
Adductors Stretch	Inner thighs	20-second static stretch following Hip Adduction exercise

Exercise	Major Muscles	Training Protocol
Abductors Stretch	Outer thighs	20-second static stretch following Hip Abduction exercise
Hip Stretch	Buttocks	20-second static stretch following Leg Press exercise
Chest Stretch	Front torso	20-second static stretch following Bench Press exercise
Upper Back Stretch	Rear torso	20-second static stretch following Seated Row exercise
Shoulder Stretch	Shoulders	20-second static stretch following Overhead Press exercise
Abdominal Stretch	Midsection	20-second static stretch following Abdominal Curl exercise
Low Back Stretch	Lower back	20-second static stretch following Low Back Extension exercise

ENDURANCE

Exercise	Warm-Up Time	Training Time	Cool-Down Time
Treadmill Walking	3 to 5 minutes easy effort	12 to 16 minutes moderate effort	3 to 5 minutes easy effort

Week Five MONDAY-WEDNESDAY-FRIDAY

Beginning this week, do breakdown training on each strength exercise for faster progress and better results (see Chapter Five).

STRENGTH

Exercise	Major Muscles	Training Protocol	Suggested Weightload
Leg Extension	Front thighs	1 set of 10 to 15 repetitions reduce weightload by 10 percent 2 more (post-fatigue) repetitions	45.0 lbs 40.0 lbs
Leg Curl	Rear thighs	1 set of 10 to 15 repetitions reduce weightload by 10 percent 2 more (post-fatigue) repetitions	45.0 lbs 40.0 lbs
Hip Adduction	Inner thighs	1 set of 10 to 15 repetitions reduce weightload by 10 percent 2 more (post-fatigue) repetitions	57.5 lbs 50.0 lbs
Hip Abduction	Outer thighs	1 set of 10 to 15 repetitions reduce weightload by 10 percent 2 more (post-fatigue) repetitions	47.5 lbs 42.5 lbs
Leg Press	Buttocks Front thighs Rear thighs	1 set of 10 to 15 repetitions reduce weightload by 10 percent 2 more (post-fatigue) repetitions	95.0 lbs 90.0 lbs
Bench Press	Chest Shoulders Rear arms	1 set of 10 to 15 repetitions reduce weightload by 10 percent 2 more (post-fatigue) repetitions	37.5 lbs 32.5 lbs
Seated Row	Upper back Front arms	1 set of 10 to 15 repetitions reduce weightload by 10 percent 2 more (post-fatigue) repetitions	52.5 lbs 47.5 lbs
Overhead Press	Shoulders Rear arms	1 set of 10 to 15 repetitions reduce weightload by 10 percent 2 more (post-fatigue) repetitions	32.5 lbs 27.5 lbs

Exercise	Major Muscles	Training Protocol	Suggested Weightload
Abdominal Curl	Midsection	1 set of 10 to 15 repetitions reduce weightload by 10 percent 2 more (post-fatigue) repetitions	45.0 lbs 40.0 lbs
Low Back Extension	Lower back	1 set of 10 to 15 repetitions reduce weightload by 10 percent 2 more (post-fatigue) repetitions	45.0 lbs 40.0 lbs

STRETCHING EXERCISE

Perform the same stretching exercises as week four, holding each stretched position for 20 seconds.

ENDURANCE

Exercise	Warm-Up Time	Training Time	Cool-Down Time
Treadmill Walking/Jogging	3 to 5 minutes slow pace	10 to 14 minutes moderate pace	3 to 5 minutes slow pace

Week Six   MONDAY-WEDNESDAY-FRIDAY

STRENGTH

Exercise	Major Muscles	Training Protocol	Suggested Weightload
Leg Extension	Front thighs	1 set of 10 to 15 repetitions reduce weightload by 10 percent 3 more (post-fatigue) repetitions	47.5 lbs 42.5 lbs
Leg Curl	Rear thighs	1 set of 10 to 15 repetitions reduce weightload by 10 percent 3 more (post-fatigue) repetitions	47.5 lbs 42.5 lbs

Exercise	Major Muscles	Training Protocol	Suggested Weightload
Hip Adduction	Inner thighs	1 set of 10 to 15 repetitions reduce weightload by 10 percent 3 more (post-fatigue) repetitions	60.0 lbs 52.5 lbs
Hip Abduction	Outer thighs	1 set of 10 to 15 repetitions reduce weightload by 10 percent 3 more (post-fatigue) repetitions	50.0 lbs 45.0 lbs
Leg Press	Buttocks Front thighs Rear thighs	1 set of 10 to 15 repetitions reduce weightload by 10 percent 3 more (post-fatigue) repetitions	100.0 lbs 90.0 lbs
Bench Press	Chest Shoulders Rear arms	1 set of 10 to 15 repetitions reduce weightload by 10 percent 3 more (post-fatigue) repetitions	40.0 lbs 35.0 lbs
Seated Row	Upper back Front arms	1 set of 10 to 15 repetitions reduce weightload by 10 percent 3 more (post-fatigue) repetitions	55.0 lbs 50.0 lbs
Overhead Press	Shoulders Rear arms	1 set of 10 to 15 repetitions reduce weightload by 10 percent 3 more (post-fatigue) repetitions	35.0 lbs 30.0 lbs
Abdominal Curl	Midsection	1 set of 10 to 15 repetitions reduce weightload by 10 percent 3 more (post-fatigue) repetitions	47.5 lbs 42.5 lbs
Low Back Extension	Lower back	1 set of 10 to 15 repetitions reduce weightload by 10 percent 3 more (post-fatigue) repetitions	47.5 lbs 42.5 lbs

STRETCHING EXERCISE

Perform the same stretching exercises as week four, holding each stretched position for 20 seconds.

Exercise	Warm-Up Time	Training Time	Cool-Down Time
Treadmill Walking/Jogging	3 to 5 minutes slow pace	12 to 16 minutes moderate pace	3 to 5 minutes slow pace

Week Seven   MONDAY-WEDNESDAY-FRIDAY

STRENGTH

Exercise	Major Muscles	Training Protocol	Suggested Weightload
Leg Extension	Front thighs	1 set of 10 to 15 repetitions reduce weightload by 10 percent 4 more (post-fatigue) repetitions	50.0 lbs 45.0 lbs
Leg Curl	Rear thighs	1 set of 10 to 15 repetitions reduce weightload by 10 percent 4 more (post-fatigue) repetitions	50.0 lbs 45.0 lbs
Hip Adduction	Inner thighs	1 set of 10 to 15 repetitions reduce weightload by 10 percent 4 more (post-fatigue) repetitions	62.5 lbs 55.0 lbs
Hip Abduction	Outer thighs	1 set of 10 to 15 repetitions reduce weightload by 10 percent 4 more (post-fatigue) repetitions	52.5 lbs 47.5 lbs
Leg Press	Buttocks Front thighs Rear thighs	1 set of 10 to 15 repetitions reduce weightload by 10 percent 4 more (post-fatigue) repetitions	105.0 lbs 95.0 lbs
Bench Press	Chest Shoulders Rear arms	1 set of 10 to 15 repetitions reduce weightload by 10 percent 4 more (post-fatigue) repetitions	42.5 lbs 37.5 lbs
Seated Row	Upper back Front arms	1 set of 10 to 15 repetitions reduce weightload by 10 percent 4 more (post-fatigue) repetitions	57.5 lbs 50.0 lbs

Exercise	Major Muscles	Training Protocol	Suggested Weightload
Overhead Press	Shoulders Rear arms	1 set of 10 to 15 repetitions reduce weightload by 10 percent 4 more (post-fatigue) repetitions	37.5 lbs 32.5 lbs
Abdominal Curl	Midsection	1 set of 10 to 15 repetitions reduce weightload by 10 percent 4 more (post-fatigue) repetitions	50.0 lbs 45.0 lbs
Low Back Extension	Lower back	1 set of 10 to 15 repetitions reduce weightload by 10 percent 4 more (post-fatigue) repetitions	50.0 lbs 45.0 lbs

STRETCHING EXERCISE

Perform the same stretching exercises as week four, holding each stretched position for 20 seconds.

ENDURANCE

Exercise	Warm-Up Time	Training Time	Cool-Down Time
Stair Climbing	3 to 5 minutes slow pace	10 to 14 minutes moderate pace	3 to 5 minutes slow pace

Week Eight   MONDAY-WEDNESDAY-FRIDAY

STRENGTH

Exercise	Major Muscles	Training Protocol	Suggested Weightload
Leg Extension	Front thighs	1 set of 10 to 15 repetitions reduce weightload by 10 percent 5 more (post-fatigue) repetitions	52.5 lbs 47.5 lbs

Exercise	Major Muscles	Training Protocol	Suggested Weightload
Leg Curl	Rear thighs	1 set of 10 to 15 repetitions reduce weightload by 10 percent 5 more (post-fatigue) repetitions	52.5 lbs 47.5 lbs
Hip Adduction	Inner thighs	1 set of 10 to 15 repetitions reduce weightload by 10 percent 5 more (post-fatigue) repetitions	65.0 lbs 57.5 lbs
Hip Abduction	Outer thighs	1 set of 10 to 15 repetitions reduce weightload by 10 percent 5 more (post-fatigue) repetitions	55.0 lbs 50.0 lbs
Leg Press	Buttocks Front thighs Rear thighs	1 set of 10 to 15 repetitions reduce weightload by 10 percent 5 more (post-fatigue) repetitions	110.0 lbs 100.0 lbs
Bench Press	Chest Shoulders Rear arms	1 set of 10 to 15 repetitions reduce weightload by 10 percent 5 more (post-fatigue) repetitions	45.0 lbs 40.0 lbs
Seated Row	Upper back Front arms	1 set of 10 to 15 repetitions reduce weightload by 10 percent 5 more (post-fatigue) repetitions	60.0 lbs 52.5 lbs
Overhead Press	Shoulders Rear arms	1 set of 10 to 15 repetitions reduce weightload by 10 percent 5 more (post-fatigue) repetitions	40.0 lbs 35.0 lbs
Abdominal Curl	Midsection	1 set of 10 to 15 repetitions reduce weightload by 10 percent 5 more (post-fatigue) repetitions	52.5 lbs 47.5 lbs
Low Back Extension	Lower back	1 set of 10 to 15 repetitions reduce weightload by 10 percent 5 more (post-fatigue) repetitions	52.5 lbs 47.5 lbs

Perform the same stretching exercises as week four, holding each stretched position for 20 seconds.

ENDURANCE

Exercise	Warm-Up Time	Training Time	Cool-Down Time
Stair Climbing	3 to 5 minutes slow pace	12 to 16 minutes moderate pace	3 to 5 minutes slow pace

This outlines two months of progressive training that will increase your physical fitness, improve your body composition, and reduce your cellulite. Strength exercise improves your muscular fitness, replaces your muscle tissue, increases your resting metabolism, decreases your body fat, and enhances your physical appearance. Endurance exercise improves your cardiovascular fitness, decreases your body fat, and enhances your physical appearance. Stretching exercise improves your flexibility fitness and enhances both your strength and endurance training.

Assuming a positive response to the anti-cellulite exercise program, you should notice major improvements in the way you look, feel, and function. After eight weeks, you should see less cellulite and experience more firmness in your hips and thighs, as well as other areas of your body.

But don't stop training. Although you may not need to train as intensely, your exercise program should become an essential component of your lifestyle if you want to maintain your physical fitness and continue to win the fight against cellulite.

10 | Results You Can Count On

BASED on our research studies, we can provide specific information about the positive physical adaptations you should experience after two months of training. Please keep in mind that these results are based solely on the exercise program, without dieting or any changes in eating habits.

The 79 Boston-area women in our initial studies at the South Shore YMCA exercise research facility represented almost every age group, with an average age of 45 years. Their exercise protocol involved three training sessions per week for a period of eight weeks. The strength training program was identical to that presented in Chapter Nine and featured the same 10 Nautilus machine exercises. These were the Hip Adduction, Hip Abduction, Leg Curl, Leg Extension, Leg Press, Bench Press, Seated Row, Overhead Press, Abdominal Curl, and Low Back Extension.

Each strength exercise was performed for one set of 10 to 15 repetitions with a challenging weightload. Whenever they could complete 15 repetitions in good form, the resistance was increased by about 5 percent for the following workout.

All repetitions were performed in a slow and controlled manner, with approximately two seconds for each lifting movement and approximately four seconds for each lowering movement. At six seconds per repetition, each exercise set required 60 to 90 seconds of continuous muscle activity. All repetitions were also performed through a full range of joint action, from the stretched muscle position to the completely contracted muscle position. The slow speed and full-range training procedures definitely enhance the exercise effectiveness.

As presented in Chapter Seven, each strengthening exercise was followed by a 20-second stretching exercise for the muscles just worked. For example, the Hip Adduction Strength exercise for the inner thigh muscles was followed by the Adductor Stretch exercise for the same muscle group. The 20-second stretches fit easily within the one-minute rest periods between successive strength exercises. Given 60 to 90 seconds to do the 10 strength exercises and a minute recovery between exercises, the total time for the strength and stretch training was typically 20 to 25 minutes.

The women's endurance exercise program was essentially the same as that presented in Chapter Eight. Each participant began at her own level of aerobic fitness and progressed gradually as her cardiovascular conditioning improved. The endurance exercises included stationary cycling, treadmill walking/jogging, and stair climbing, but other aerobic activities such as elliptical striding, cross-country ski simulation, and rowing should be equally effective. Including warm-up and cool-down, the total time for the endurance training was typically 20 to 25 minutes.

Exercise Program Results

The results from our 45-minute combined strength, stretch, and endurance exercise program were very encouraging. On average, the women who did not change their eating pattern lost 3.2 pounds of fat and replaced 1.7 pounds of muscle for a major improvement in their body composition and physical appearance.

Much of the fat loss occurred in the hip and thigh areas, which represented the main fat storage areas for most of our program participants. We assessed the hip/buttocks girth before and after the two-month training period. The average reduction in this circumference measurement was 1.0 inches, indicating a large fat loss in the hip/buttocks as well as a smaller dress/pant size.

With the use of ultrasound technology (sonar), we were also able to assess the thickness of the subcutaneous fat layer in the women's thighs. This is the fat layer between the thigh muscles and the skin that is largely responsible for the soft and lumpy cellulite look. On average, this surrounding fat layer was reduced in thickness by 1.4 millimeters, which represents a significant amount of fat loss in the women's thighs.

Muscle was added where muscle was needed, namely to the leg-shaping and figure-defining muscles of the thighs. These should be the largest, strongest, and most attractive muscles in the human body, but a sedentary lifestyle renders the once-firm thigh muscles weak and flabby. Without question, the most important aspect of the cellulite reduction program is to rebuild and reshape the long thigh muscles.

Our ultrasound measurements revealed a 1.7-millimeter increase in thigh muscle thickness over the eight-week exercise period. This was undoubtedly our most encouraging finding, indicating that the women were remodeling their muscles to provide shapely thighs and a solid base for the overlying fat layer. With more muscle for a higher metabolic rate and a firmer underlying foundation, continued fat loss and cellulite reduction is almost certain. In addition to the body composition benefits, the women experienced an average strength increase of 49 percent for enhanced physical capacity and personal functionality.

Three Times More Fat Loss

After determining that the exercise program alone is highly effective for reducing fat and replacing muscle, we added a nutrition component to see if even better results could be attained during the eight-week training period. The next chapter presents the general and specific guidelines for incorporating this purposeful nutrition plan into your cellulite reduction program. And if fat loss is a major objective, then you definitely should follow these tested dietary recommendations.

As you will see in Table 10.1, the women who did both the exercise program and the nutrition plan lost 7.9 pounds of weight compared to 1.5 pounds for those who did only the exercise program. Although the muscle gain was similar for both groups (1.2 pounds vs. 1.7 pounds), the nutrition plan participants lost almost three times more fat than the nondieters (9.1 pounds vs. 3.2 pounds). They lost

Table 10.1

Comparative results for women who did both the exercise program and nutrition plan with women who did the exercise program only.

Fitness Parameter	Exercise Program Only	Exercise Program and Nutrition Plan
Weight loss	−1.5 lbs	−7.9 lbs
Fat loss	−3.2 lbs	−9.1 lbs
Muscle gain	+ 1.7 lbs	+ 1.2 lbs
Body composition change	4.9 lbs	10.3 lbs
Hip girth reduction	−1.0 ins	−1.8 ins
Strength increase	+49.3 %	+46.0 %

more than one pound of fat per week, which represents an excellent and sustainable rate of progression toward a lower and healthier body weight.

In terms of body composition, the nutrition plan participants improved twice as much as their peers who performed only the exercise program (10.3 pounds vs. 4.9 pounds). The exercise and diet group also had almost two times the hip girth reduction as the exercise only group (1.8 inches vs. 1.0 inches).

Finally, the additional fat loss did not negatively affect strength gains or functional capacity in the women who ate fewer calories. The diet and exercise group experienced a 46 percent increase in muscle strength compared to a 49 percent strength gain in the exercise only group.

If you desire better and faster results, be sure to include the Purposeful Nutrition Plan in your cellulite program. In all fairness, the women who consistently followed the nutritional guidelines made the most improvement, whereas those who took an on-again/off-again dietary approach had more modest results. Our most compliant participants lost 13 to 14 pounds of unattractive fat while concurrently replacing 1 to 2 pounds of shapely muscle, for a 15-pound improvement in their body composition and personal appearance. Because you will be hard-pressed to find a better balanced and more successful nutrition plan, we strongly recommend that you follow the dietary guidelines closely and consistently in conjunction with your exercise program.

The Critical Measure of Success

As impressive as these positive body composition changes are, a key question needed to be addressed, and the study participants were the only ones who could answer it. The key question, of course, was how did the exercise program impact their cellulite situation? Did it have any affect on their cellulite appearance, and if so, how large was the improvement?

Unfortunately, there is no objective means for measuring cellulite. We simply don't have cellulite meters or lumpiness indicators. Basically, we know cellulite when we see it, and we must subjectively determine if it is looking better or getting worse. To obtain honest opinions, we gave all the women a written questionnaire on which they wrote anonymous responses to this and other questions regarding their perceptions of the exercise program components and outcomes. We trust that the responses we received represented the participants' true feelings regarding the program results.

Remarkably, 70 percent of the participants reported that they had a *lot less cellulite* after completing the exercise program. The remaining 30 percent reported that they had *less cellulite* at the end of the training period. That is, 100 percent of the women felt the program was beneficial and accomplished the main objective of improving their cellulite problem. Be assured, all the participants saw some cellulite reduction, and almost three-quarters of the participants indicated major cellulite reduction.

Participants' Perceptions of the Program

To attain a more complete picture of the women's perceptions about the exercise program, our written questionnaire requested feedback on all of the program components. The participants responded to each of the following statements using a 5.0 point scale, with 1.0 representing the lowest rating and 5.0 representing the highest rating.

statement 1 | The exercise program improved my muscle strength.
Average Rating: 4.6

statement 2 | The exercise program improved my cardiovascular endurance.
Average Rating: 4.4

| statement 3 | The exercise program improved my joint flexibility. |
| | **Average Rating:** 4.1 |

| statement 4 | The exercise program improved my body composition. |
| | **Average Rating:** 4.3 |

| statement 5 | The exercise program improved my physical appearance. |
| | **Average Rating:** 3.8 |

| statement 6 | The exercise program improved my cellulite problem. |
| | **Average Rating:** 3.9 |

| statement 7 | The exercise program improved my self-confidence. |
| | **Average Rating:** 4.5 |

| statement 8 | The exercise program was a positive and productive experience. |
| | **Average Rating:** 4.8 |

| statement 9 | The exercise program was safe, effective, and efficient. |
| | **Average Rating:** 4.8 |

These nine aspects of the anti-cellulite exercise program averaged 4.4 on a 5.0-point rating scale, indicating that the participants were very pleased with both the training process and the training products. Apparently, these women had positive exercise experiences that enabled them to reduce cellulite and enhance their personal appearance. We believe the same exercise program that worked so well for them can produce similar effects in women of all ages, shapes, and sizes.

Summary

The 79 middle-age women who participated in our initial cellulite-reduction research studies experienced excellent results from their 45-minute exercise program that included strength training, stretching, and aerobic activity. After two months of training, those who did not diet lost 3.2 pounds of fat and added 1.7 pounds of muscle for a major improvement in their body composition and physical appearance. They also reduced their hip size by 1.0 inch and increased their muscle strength by 49 percent. The women who combined the nutrition plan with their exercise program replaced almost as much muscle (1.2 pounds), but lost almost three times as much fat (9.1 pounds), for a 7.9-pound weight loss and a 10.3-pound improvement in their body composition and physical appearance. Most important, 70 percent of the participants reported that they had a lot less cellulite after completing the exercise program, and the other 30 percent reported less cellulite. These personal perceptions were confirmed by ultrasound measurements of their thighs, which showed a 1.4-millimeter decrease in the fat layer and a 1.7-millimeter increase in the muscle layer. In addition, all the women stated that the exercise program was a positive and productive experience that improved their muscle strength, joint flexibility, cardiovascular endurance, and self-confidence.

11 | Purposeful Nutrition Plan

Our initial research on cellulite reduction focused solely on the exercise components, namely strength training, aerobic activity, and stretching. We did not provide a diet plan or nutritional guidelines for reducing body weight. We wanted to determine whether our exercise program was effective for replacing muscle and reducing fat sufficiently to improve the participants' cellulite situation.

The basic exercise program worked extremely well, with 30 percent of the women reporting less cellulite and 70 percent of the women reporting a lot less cellulite. Nevertheless, the muscle gain (1.7 pounds) and fat loss (3.2 pounds) in our first studies combined for a relatively small change in body weight (1.5 pounds). Obviously, we should be able to attain greater fat reduction with reasonable calorie restrictions in a balanced nutrition plan. However, we are also aware that too little food intake can limit muscle replacement, and muscle rebuilding is the absolutely essential element in our cellulite reduction program.

We have worked hard, with assistance from registered dieticians and nutrition professors, to develop a practical eating protocol that accelerates fat loss without attenuating muscle development. Our final product, known as the Purposeful Nutrition Plan, is completely consistent with the USDA Food Guide Pyramid yet offers numerous options for addressing individual needs and accommodating personal preferences. Our research participants who combined the Purposeful Nutrition Plan with their exercise program lost up to 14 pounds of fat and still added 1 to 2 pounds of muscle during the eight-week training period.

USDA Food Guide Pyramid

As shown in Figure 11.1, the Food Guide Pyramid provides a basic framework for categorizing food groups and selecting serving quantities.

The foods at the base of the Food Guide Pyramid should be most prominent in a healthy diet, and include grains, rice, cereals, breads, and pasta. These staple foods provide complex carbohydrates for energy, as well as important vitamins, minerals, and fiber. The second level of the Pyramid features fruits and vegetables, most of which are excellent sources of carbohydrates, vitamins, minerals, and fiber. The next level of recommended food groups is divided between protein-rich selections from meat and dairy sources. These foods include beef, pork, lamb, poultry, fish, milk, yogurt, cheese, eggs, and nuts, and collectively supply calcium, iron, and zinc as well as all the essential amino acids (proteins). The Pyramid peak is limited to foods that are high in calories and low in nutrients, such as fats, sweets, and oils.

The amount of food you eat is determined by your energy requirements and varies widely depending on your age, gender, body weight, muscle mass, activity level, and metabolic factors. Based on your daily calorie requirements, the recommended number of servings from each food group will be different but proportional. Table 11.1 presents suggested food group servings for three common

Figure 11.1

U.S. Department of Agriculture Food Guide Pyramid.

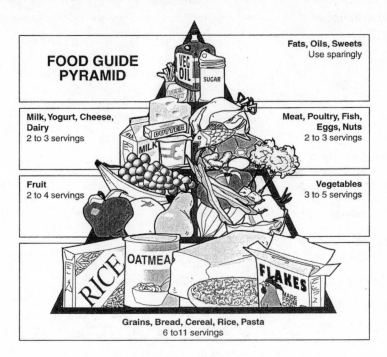

categories of daily calorie consumption. If your daily calorie needs fall between or outside these examples, simply estimate your appropriate food group servings accordingly.

Serving Sizes

Knowing how many servings to eat from each food group category is certainly important for proper nutritional balance, as well as total calorie consumption. However, you should also understand how much food constitutes a serving so you do not undereat or overeat a particular food group. Table 11.1 provides practical information on standard serving sizes for each food group category.

Although almost all nutritionists and medical professionals advise against

Table 11.1

Recommended number of food group servings for three common levels of daily calorie consumption.

	Daily Calorie Consumption Categories		
	Group One (1,600 Cal.)	**Group Two** (2,200 Cal.)	**Group Three** (2,800 Cal.)
Bread and grain group servings	6	9	11
Vegetable group servings	3	4	5
Fruit group servings	2	3	4
Milk group servings	2–3	2–3	2–3
Meat group servings	2–3	2–3	2–3
Notes:	*Suggested for many sedentary women and some older adults.*	*Suggested for most children, teenage girls, active women, and many sedentary men.*	*Suggested for teenage boys, many active men, and some very active women.*

high-protein diets (such as the Atkins Diet), you may prefer a nutrition program that features a higher percentage of protein-rich foods. If so, you may still use our recommended nutrition plan effectively. Simply reduce the number of bread and grain group servings by the additional number of milk and meat group servings.

Because there are so many variations even within the basic food groups, please consider some suggestions for making heart-healthy and weight-wise selections.

Table 11.2

Recommended serving sizes for the various food group categories.

Food Group	Examples of a Single Serving
Breads and grains	1 slice bread $1/2$ cup cooked pasta $1/2$ cup cooked rice $1/2$ bagel 1 ounce cereal
Vegetables	1 cup leafy raw vegetables $1/2$ cup nonleafy, chopped raw vegetables $1/2$ cup cooked vegetables
Fruits	1 whole fruit $3/4$ cup fruit juice $1/2$ cup canned fruit
Milk products	1 cup milk $1/2$ cup ice cream or frozen yogurt 8 ounces yogurt 2 ounces cheese
Meats	3 ounces lean meat, poultry, or fish 1 egg $1/2$ cup dry beans 2 tablespoons peanut butter

Breads and Grains

Whole-grain breads, cereals, and pastas and brown rice are higher in fiber than popular alternatives, such as enriched white flour products. Eating high-fiber foods may assist in stabilizing blood sugar and help in reducing food cravings.

Vegetables

Use several types of vegetables to obtain a desirable nutritional balance. Dark green leafy vegetables are more nutrient-dense than popular iceberg lettuce. To minimize loss of vitamins and minerals, eat raw, steamed, stir-fried, or microwaved vegetables. Keep chopped vegetables in the refrigerator for healthy snack foods.

Fruits

Like vegetables, fresh fruits make excellent low-fat snacks. Although higher in calories, dried fruits are a very good source of fiber, vitamins, and minerals. Fruit juices are superb all-purpose beverages, although they lack fiber and may have higher sugar content than equal amounts of raw fruit.

Meats

Leaner white meats such as fish, chicken breast, and pork tenderloin are preferable to fatter dark meats. Always remove the skin and trim all visible fat before cooking meats. If you use canned tuna, keep in mind that water-packed varieties have much less fat than oil-packed alternatives. All-natural peanut butters have less sugar and healthier fats than other types. Be aware that beans and legumes also constitute excellent protein sources.

Fats

Fats are an essential component of a healthy diet but should be eaten sparingly. Because fats contain more than twice as many calories per gram as carbohydrates and proteins, reducing fat intake is the best way to cut back your daily calorie consumption. Be aware that large quantities of hidden fats are present in most baked goods, salad dressings, processed foods, and food toppings.

Water

Because water is essential for all body functions, it is the most important nutrient, even though it contains no calories, proteins, carbohydrates, fats, or vitamins. You should drink at least eight cups of water throughout the day, especially before, during, and after exercise sessions. If you don't enjoy drinking plain water, try adding lemon or lime slices for flavor. In our experience, drinking extra water provides extra benefits, not only making the skin look better, but also enhancing muscle development and taking the edge off your appetite. Drinking cold water also burns additional calories, as it must be warmed to body temperature. Although plain water is fine, you may substitute flavored varieties, vitamin/mineral-enhanced waters, or similar noncaloric beverages if you prefer.

Weight Management Menu Plan

Our weight management menu plan is not a diet in the traditional sense. Rather, it represents a purposeful and practical lifestyle change that can be continued indefinitely because it is individualized to meet your nutritional needs and address your food group preferences. The weight management menu plan offers three daily calorie consumption categories that are consistent with those in the Food Guide Pyramid. Depending on your physical characteristics and weight loss objectives, you may choose the 1,600-calorie, 2,200-calorie, or 2,800-calorie daily menu plan (see Table 11.1) Generally speaking, large-framed women may begin with the 2,800-calorie plan, medium-framed women may begin with the 2,200-calorie plan, and small-framed women may begin with the 1,600-calorie plan. Of course, your calorie plan should be lower than your current daily caloric intake to facilitate fat loss. However, we do not recommend reducing more than 500 calories a day below your present level, as you need sufficient energy to exercise effectively. A 500-calorie-per-day deficit should result in a 1-pound per week fat loss, independent from your exercise program.

Basically, the menu plan is a simple means for tracking your daily servings in each of the food groups. Just check off each food item that you eat in the appropriate category. In addition, the menu plan presents 12 sample daily eating programs, as well as eight new main course recipes you may want to try. The recipes of the week are designed to please you and your family and include chicken, fish, turkey, pork, beef, pasta, and vegetarian meals.

The goal is to develop your own healthy meals using the recommended food group servings to stay within your desired calorie range. Of course, you have to keep a careful eye on portion sizes or you can easily exceed your caloric expectations.

Sample Menus

The 12 daily menus present sample foods for breakfast, lunch, dinner, and snacks. You may follow the menus exactly, or you may substitute similar food items. For example, you can substitute six ounces grape juice for six ounces orange juice, one-half cup corn for one-half cup peas, three ounces chicken for three ounces pork, one English muffin for two slices wheat bread, and so on. Just make certain the food item you substitute has approximately the same number of calories as the recommended food item.

If you want to eat approximately 1,600 calories a day, use the **Group One** column for portion/calorie recommendations. If you plan to eat approximately 2,200 calories a day, use the **Group Two** column for portion/calorie recommendations. If you require about 2,800 calories a day, use the **Group Three** column for portion/calorie recommendations. If your daily calorie goal is between these guidelines, adjust the portion sizes accordingly. Regardless of your food intake, be sure to drink plenty of water all day long for enhanced weight loss and cellulite reduction results.

Menu One

Food	Group One	Group Two	Group Three
	portion/calories	portion/calories	portion/calories
BREAKFAST			
Waffles	2 each/174	2 each/174	2 each/174
Butter	1 tbsp./102	1 tbsp./102	1 tbsp./102
Peanut butter	2 tbsp./188	2 tbsp./188	2 tbsp./188
Banana	1 small/93	1 small/93	1 small/93
Skim milk	8 oz./86	8 oz./86	8 oz./86
Peach	—	—	1 each/42
SNACK			
Fat-free wheat crackers	—	16 each/160	16 each/160
LUNCH			
Tuna fish	2 oz./73	3 oz./110	3 oz./110
Mayo	1 tbsp./100	1 tbsp./100	1 tbsp./100
Wheat bread	2 slices/130	2 slices/130	2 slices/130
Lettuce and tomato	—	1/2 cup/10	1/2 cup/10
Skim milk	8 oz./86	8 oz./86	8 oz./86
Apple	—	1 each/80	1 each/80

Menu One (Continued)

Food	Group One portion/calories	Group Two portion/calories	Group Three portion/calories
SNACK			
Pear	1 each/100	1 each/100	1 each/100
DINNER			
Skim milk	8 oz./86	8 oz./86	8 oz./86
Pasta	1 cup/197	1 cup/197	1 1/2 cups/296
Tomato sauce	1/2 cup/71	1/2 cup/71	1 cup/142
Zucchini	1/2 cup/14	1/2 cup/14	1/2 cup/14
Ground turkey	2 oz./84	2 oz./84	3 oz./126
Garlic bread	—	1 slice/82	2 slices/161
Made with butter	—	1 tbsp./102	1 tbsp./102
SNACK			
Celery sticks	1/2 cup/10	1/2 cup/10	1/2 cup/10

Menu Two

Food	Group One portion/calories	Group Two portion/calories	Group Three portion/calories
BREAKFAST			
Fat-free vanilla yogurt	8 oz./206	8 oz./206	8 oz./206
Peach	1/40	1/40	1/40
Granola cereal	1 oz./129	2 oz./257	3 oz./386
Orange juice	—	—	6 oz./86
LUNCH			
Wheat bread	2 slices/130	2 slices/130	2 slices/130
Chicken	2 oz./112	3 oz./168	3 oz./168
Skim milk	8 oz./86	8 oz./86	8 oz./86
Mixed vegetables	1/2 cup/54	1 cup/107	1 1/2 cups/161
Mayo	—	—	1 tbsp./100

Menu Two (Continued)

Food	Group One portion/calories	Group Two portion/calories	Group Three portion/calories
SNACK			
English muffin	1 each/133	1 each/133	1 each/133
Butter	1 tbsp./102	1 tbsp./102	1 tbsp./102
DINNER			
Skim milk	8 oz./86	8 oz./86	8 oz./86
Roast turkey	3 oz./161	3 oz./161	4 oz./215
Bread stuffing	1/2 cup/178	1 cup/356	1 cup/356
Green beans	1/2 cup/19	1/2 cup/19	1/2 cup/19
Corn	1/2 cup/66	1/2 cup/66	1/2 cup/66
SNACK			
Fruit cocktail	1/2 cup/54	1 cup/108	1 cup/108
Fat-free crackers	—	8 each/80	16 each/160

Menu Three

Food	Group One portion/calories	Group Two portion/calories	Group Three portion/calories
BREAKFAST			
English muffin	1 each/133	1 each/133	1 each/133
Fat-free vanilla yogurt	8 oz./206	8 oz./206	8 oz./206
Orange juice	6 oz./86	12 oz./172	12 oz./172
Low-fat granola	—	2 oz./220	3 oz./330
LUNCH			
Hummus	1/2 cup/208	1/2 cup/208	1 cup/416
Pita bread	1–6"/165	1–6"/165	1–6"/165
Nonfat frozen yogurt	1 cup/191	1 cup/191	1 cup/191
Strawberries	1/2 cup/25	1/2 cup/25	1 cup/50
Angelfood cake	—	—	1/6 of cake/146

Menu Three (Continued)

Food	Group One portion/calories	Group Two portion/calories	Group Three portion/calories
DINNER			
Skim milk	1 cup/86	1 cup/86	1 cup/86
Baked chicken	4 oz./223	5 oz./279	5 oz./279
Corn	$1/2$ cup/66	1 cup/132	1 cup/132
Peas	—	—	$1/2$ cup/62
Oven-fried sweet potatoes	1 cup/176	1 cup/176	1 cup/176
SNACK			
Chips Ahoy® cookies	4 each/213	4 each/213	4 each/213

Menu Four

Food	Group One portion/calories	Group Two portion/calories	Group Three portion/calories
BREAKFAST			
Grapefruit	$1/2$/60 each	$1/2$/60 each	$1/2$/60 each
Bagel	1 small/195	1 large/303	1 large/303
Butter	—	1 tbsp./102	1 tbsp./102
Nonfat vanilla yogurt	8 oz./206	8 oz./206	8 oz./206
LUNCH			
Chicken salad			
Chicken breast	2 oz./112	3 oz./168	4 oz./224
Celery	$1/2$ cup/10	$1/2$ cup/10	$1/2$ cup/10
Mayo	1 tbsp./100	1 tbsp./100	1 tbsp./100
Bulky roll	1 each/152	1 each/152	1 each/152
Skim milk	1 cup/86	1 cup/86	1 cup/86
Side salad	—	—	1 cup/22
Ranch dressing	—	—	1 tbsp./60

Menu Four (Continued)

Food	Group One portion/calories	Group Two portion/calories	Group Three portion/calories
SNACK			
Banana	1 small/93	1 large/125	1 large/125
DINNER			
Skim milk	1 cup/86	1 cup/86	1 cup/86
Pork stir-fry			
Pork	3 oz./206	3 oz./206	3 oz./206
Red and green peppers	1/2 cup/20	1 cup/40	1 cup/40
Broccoli	1/2 cup/10	1/2 cup/10	1/2 cup/10
Peanut oil	1 tbsp./119	1 tbsp./119	1 tbsp./119
Brown rice	1 cup/218	1 cup/218	1 1/2 cup/327
SNACK			
Graham crackers	—	5 each/75	10 each/150
Apple juice	—	—	6 oz./87

Menu Five

Food	Group One portion/calories	Group Two portion/calories	Group Three portion/calories
BREAKFAST			
Orange juice	6 oz./86	6 oz./86	12 oz./172
Honey Bunches of Oats® cereal	2 oz./223	2 oz./223	3 oz./335
Skim milk	1 cup/86	1 cup/86	1 cup/86
LUNCH			
Turkey	2 oz./107	3 oz./161	3 oz./161
Swiss cheese	1 oz./95	1 oz./95	1 oz./95
Tomatoes	1/4 cup/9	1/4 cup/9	1/4 cup/9
Roll	1 each/152	1 each/152	1 each/152
Mayo	—	1 tbsp./100	1 tbsp./100
Grapes	1/2 cup/30	1/2 cup/30	1/2 cup/30
Vegetable juice	6 oz./34	12 oz./68	12 oz./68

Menu Five (Continued)

Food	Group One portion/calories	Group Two portion/calories	Group Three portion/calories
LUNCH (Continued)			
Carrot sticks	1/2 cup/28	1/2 cup/28	1 cup/56
Ranch dressing	1 tbsp./60	1 tbsp./60	1 tbsp./60
SNACK			
Fat-free vanilla yogurt	8 oz./206	8 oz./206	8 oz./206
Low-fat granola	—	2 oz./220	3 oz./330
DINNER			
Chicken breast	3 oz./168	3 oz./168	4 oz./224
Salsa	1/4 cup/18	1/4 cup/18	1/4 cup/18
Cheddar cheese	1 oz./114	1 oz./114	1 oz./114
Spanish rice	1 cup/216	1 1/2 cups/324	1 1/2 cups/324
SNACK			
Apple	—	1 each/80	1 each/80

Menu Six

Food	Group One portion/calories	Group Two portion/calories	Group Three portion/calories
BREAKFAST			
English muffin	1 each/133	1 each/133	1 each/133
Butter	—	1 tbsp./102	1 tbsp./102
Fat-free vanilla yogurt	8 oz./206	8 oz./206	8 oz./206
Raisins	1/4 cup/107	1/4 cup/107	1/4 cup/107
Low-fat granola	2 oz./220	3 oz./330	4 oz./440
LUNCH			
Grilled cheese			
Wheat bread	2 slices/130	2 slices/130	2 slices/130
American cheese	2 oz./186	2 oz./186	2 oz./186
Tomatoes	1/2 cup/19	1/2 cup/19	1/2 cup/19
Butter	1 tbsp./102	1 tbsp./102	1 tbsp./102

Menu Six (Continued)

Food	Group One portion/calories	Group Two portion/calories	Group Three portion/calories
LUNCH (Continued)			
Mixed green salad	—	1 cup/9	2 cup/18
Chickpeas	—	—	1 cup/286
Cranberry juice	6 oz./97	12 oz./194	12 oz./194
SNACK			
Graham crackers	—	12 each/180	18 each/270
Peanut butter	—	1 tbsp./94	1 tbsp./94
DINNER			
Haddock	5 oz./169	6 oz./203	6 oz./203
Baked potato	1 each/133	1 each/133	1 each/133
Stuffed with broccoli	1/2 cup/26	1/2 cup/26	1/2 cup/26
Fat-free shredded cheese	2 oz./81	2 oz./81	2 oz./81
Honeydew melon	—	—	1/2 cup/30

Menu Seven

Food	Group One portion/calories	Group Two portion/calories	Group Three portion/calories
BREAKFAST			
Bagel	1 small/195	1 large/303	1 large/303
Butter	—	1 tbsp./102	1 tbsp./102
Cranberry juice	6 oz./97	12 oz./194	12 oz./194
Banana	—	—	1 small/92
LUNCH			
Tuna	2 oz./73	2 oz./73	3 oz./110
Mayo	1 tbsp./100	1 tbsp./100	1 tbsp./100
Wheat bread	2 slices/130	2 slices/130	2 slices/130
Lettuce	1/2 cup/3	1/2 cup/3	1 cup/6
Tomatoes	1/4 cup/10	1/4 cup/10	1/2 cup/20
Apple	1 each/80	1 each/80	1 each/80

Menu Seven (Continued)

Food	Group One portion/calories	Group Two portion/calories	Group Three portion/calories
LUNCH (Continued)			
Skim milk	8 oz./86	8 oz./86	8 oz./86
Graham cracker	—	—	12 each/180
DINNER			
Ham—low sodium	3 oz./155	4 oz./206	4 oz./206
Squash	1/2 cup/18	1 cup/36	1 cup/36
Baked potato	1 each/133	1 each/133	1 each/133
Butter	1 tbsp./102	1 tbsp./102	1 tbsp./102
Skim milk	8 oz./86	8 oz./86	8 oz./86
SNACK			
Fat-free vanilla yogurt	8 oz./206	8 oz./206	8 oz./206
Grape-Nuts® cereal	2 oz./204	3 oz./306	3 oz./306

Menu Eight

Food	Group One portion/calories	Group Two portion/calories	Group Three portion/calories
BREAKFAST			
Cheerios® cereal	2 oz./207	2 oz./207	2 oz./207
Skim milk	8 oz./86	8 oz./86	8 oz./86
Apple juice	6 oz./87	6 oz./87	12 oz./174
Bagel	1/2 small/98	1 small/195	1 large/303
Cream cheese	1 oz./99	1 oz./99	2 oz./198
Sugar	—	—	1 tbsp./46
SNACK			
Orange	1 each/70	1 each/70	1 each/70
LUNCH			
Wheat bread	2 slices/130	2 slices/130	2 slices/130
Turkey breast	2 oz./107	3 oz./161	3 oz./161
Mayo	1 tbsp./100	1 tbsp./100	1 tbsp./100

Menu Eight (Continued)

Food	Group One portion/calories	Group Two portion/calories	Group Three portion/calories
LUNCH (Continued)			
Skim milk	8 oz./86	8 oz./86	8 oz./86
Side salad	—	1 cup/22	1 cup/22
Ranch salad dressing	—	1 tbsp./60	2 tbsp./120
Apple	—	1 each/80	1 each/80
SNACK			
Celery and carrot sticks	1/2 cup/18	1 cup/36	1 cup/36
Graham crackers	—	4 each/60	4 each/60
DINNER			
Skim milk	8 oz./86	8 oz./86	8 oz./86
Chicken breast	3 oz./168	3 oz./168	4 oz./224
Dinner roll	1 each/107	1 each/107	1 each/107
Brown rice	—	1/2 cup/109	1/2 cup/109
Green beans	1/2 cup/20	—	1/2 cup/20
Corn	1/2 cup/66	1/2 cup/66	1/2 cup/66
Butter	—	1 tbsp./102	2 tbsp./204

Menu Nine

Food	Group One portion/calories	Group Two portion/calories	Group Three portion/calories
BREAKFAST			
Special K® cereal	2 oz./210	2 oz./210	4 oz./420
Skim milk	1 cup/86	1 cup/86	1 cup/86
Apple juice	12 oz./175	12 oz./175	12 oz./175
LUNCH			
Wheat bread	2 slices/130	2 slices/130	2 slices/130
Ham	2 oz./103	3 oz./155	3 oz./155
American cheese	2 oz./186	2 oz./186	2 oz./186
Lettuce	—	1/2 cup/3	1 cup/6

Menu Nine (Continued)

Food	Group One portion/calories	Group Two portion/calories	Group Three portion/calories
LUNCH (Continued)			
Tomatoes	—	1/4 cup/10	1/2 cup/19
Banana	—	1 small/93	1 large/125
SNACK			
Fat-free crackers	8 each/80	16 each/160	16 each/160
DINNER			
Skim milk	1 cup/86	1 cup/86	1 cup/86
Haddock	3 oz./101	3 oz./101	4 oz./135
Butter	—	1 tbsp./102	1 tbsp./102
Bread crumbs	—	1/2 cup/220	1/2 cup/220
Baked potato	1 each/133	1 each/133	1 each/133
Mixed veggies	1 cup/107	1 cup/107	1 cup/107
SNACK			
Bagel	1/2 small/98	1 small/195	1 small/195
Butter	1 tbsp./102	—	1 tbsp./102

Menu Ten

Food	Group One portion/calories	Group Two portion/calories	Group Three portion/calories
BREAKFAST			
Scrambled eggs			
Whole egg	1 each/75	2 each/150	2 each/150
American cheese	1 oz./93	1 oz./93	1 oz./93
Skim milk	4 oz./43	4 oz./43	4 oz./43
Orange juice	6 oz./86	12 oz./172	12 oz./172
English muffin	1 each/133	1 each/133	2 each/266
Butter	—	1 tbsp./102	1 tbsp./102

Menu Ten (Continued)

Food	Group One portion/calories	Group Two portion/calories	Group Three portion/calories
LUNCH			
Tuna fish	3 oz./109	3 oz./109	4 oz./145
Wheat bread	2 slices/130	2 slices/130	2 slices/130
Mayo	1 tbsp./100	1 tbsp./100	1 tbsp./100
Celery sticks	1/2 cup/10	1 cup/20	1 cup/20
Peanut butter	2 tbsp./188	2 tbsp./188	2 tbsp./188
Skim milk	1 cup/86	1 cup/86	1 cup/86
SNACK			
Peach	1 each/40	1 each/40	1 each/40
DINNER			
Pasta salad			
Pasta	1 cup/197	2 cup/394	2 cup/394
Red and green peppers	1/2 cup/12	1/2 cup/12	1 cup/24
Celery and cucumber	1/2 cup/8	1/2 cup/8	1/2 cup/8
Fat-free Italian dressing	1 tbsp./10	1 tbsp./10	1 tbsp./10
SNACK			
Fat-free vanilla yogurt	8 oz./206	8 oz./206	8 oz./206
Low-fat granola	—	1 oz./128	1 oz./128
Raisins	—	—	1/4 cup/107

Menu Eleven

Food	Group One portion/calories	Group Two portion/calories	Group Three portion/calories
BREAKFAST			
Grape-Nuts® cereal	1 oz./102	2 oz./204	2 oz./204
Cheerios® cereal	2 oz./207	2 oz./207	3 oz./311
Skim milk	1 cup/86	1 cup/86	1 cup/86
Wheat toast	—	—	1 slice/65
Orange	1 each/70	1 each/70	1 each/70
Butter	—	—	1 tbsp./102

Menu Eleven (Continued)

Food	Group One portion/calories	Group Two portion/calories	Group Three portion/calories
LUNCH			
Wheat bread	2 slices/130	2 slices/130	2 slices/130
Tuna	2 oz./73	2 oz./73	3 oz./110
Mayo	—	1 tbsp./100	1 tbsp./100
Celery, chopped	1/4 cup/5	1/4 cup/5	1/4 cup/5
Carrots, chopped	—	—	1/4 cup/14
Lettuce	1/2 cup/3	1/2 cup/3	1/2 cup/3
Tomato	—	—	1/2 cup/19
Apple juice	6 oz./87	6 oz./87	12 oz./174
SNACK			
Fat-free crackers	—	12 each/120	12 each/120
Peanut butter	—	2 tbsp./188	2 tbsp./188
DINNER			
Salmon, grilled	3 oz./118	3 oz./118	3 oz./118
Tossed salad	1 cup/22	1 cup/22	1 cup/22
Olive oil	1 tbsp./119	1 tbsp./119	1 tbsp./119
Broccoli	1/2 cup/26	1 cup/52	1 cup/52
Dinner roll	1 each/107	1 each/107	1 each/107
Vanilla ice cream	1/2 cup/133	1/2 cup/133	1/2 cup/133
SNACK			
Fat-free vanilla yogurt	8 oz./206	8 oz./206	8 oz./206
Apple	—	1 each/80	1 each/80

Menu Twelve

Food	Group One portion/calories	Group Two portion/calories	Group Three portion/calories
BREAKFAST			
Hard-boiled egg	1 each/75	1 each/75	1 each/75
Wheat toast	2 slices/130	2 slices/130	2 slices/130

Menu Twelve (Continued)

Food	Group One portion/calories	Group Two portion/calories	Group Three portion/calories
BREAKFAST (Continued)			
Butter	1 tbsp./102	1 tbsp./102	1 tbsp./102
Grapefruit juice	6 oz./70	12 oz./140	12 oz./140
Fat-free vanilla yogurt	8 oz./206	8 oz./206	8 oz./206
LUNCH			
Three-bean salad	1 cup/160	1 cup/160	1½ cup/204
Skim milk	1 cup/86	1 cup/86	1 cup/86
Pita bread	1-6"/165	1-6"/165	1-6"/165
Side salad	1 cup/22	2 cups/44	2 cups/44
Ranch salad dressing	1 tbsp./60	1 tbsp./60	1 tbsp./60
Cantaloupe	½ cup/29	½ cup/29	1 cup/57
SNACK			
Bagel	—	—	½ small/98
Cream cheese	—	—	1 oz./99
DINNER			
Stir-fry			
Rice	1 cup/218	1½ cups/327	2 cups/436
Chicken breast	2 oz./112	3 oz./168	3 oz./168
Red, green pepper, and onion	1 cup/24	1 cup/24	1½ cups/36
Skim milk	8 oz./86	8 oz./86	8 oz./86
SNACK			
Vanilla wafers	—	10 each/190	10 each/190

Main Course Recipes

Pork Chops Dijon

YIELD 4 SERVINGS

The pork chop would count as a meat. The size of the chop would determine how many ounces it would count as.

1 tbsp olive oil

4 ¾-inch-thick pork chops, trimmed of fat

2 tbsps vinegar

1 tsp Dijon mustard

¼ cup low-fat milk

1. In a large skillet, place olive oil, add pork chops, and slowly cook over low heat, turning occasionally for about 30–35 minutes or until brown and tender.

2. Remove from skillet and keep warm. Increase the heat and de-glaze the skillet by adding vinegar and stirring well, scrapping up any brown bits.

3. Stir in mustard first, then milk and simmer, stirring, for 2–3 minutes. Serve over or under pork chops.

Cucumber Salad

YIELD 8 SERVINGS

A ½-cup serving would count as 1 serving of the vegetable group.

1 cup nonfat plain yogurt	1 tsp finely minced fresh
1 clove garlic, crushed	gingerroot
½ cup sliced scallions	2 medium cucumbers, peeled and
⅛ tsp black pepper	thinly sliced

1. Mix together yogurt, garlic, scallions, black pepper, and gingerroot in a serving bowl. Add cucumbers and toss.

2. Chill for one hour before serving.

Herb-Baked Scrod

YIELD 4 SERVINGS

The fish would count toward the meat group. The size of the fillet would determine how many ounces it would count as.

4 fillets (about 2 lbs)	¼ tsp Mrs. Dash herb and
½ cup bread crumbs	garlic seasoning
¼ cup grated low-fat	1 tbsp minced fresh parsley
Parmesan cheese	½ cup fat-free mayo
¼ tsp dried dill weed	1 tbsp lemon juice

1. Rinse fish and dry between paper towels.

2. In pie plate, combine bread crumbs, Parmesan cheese, dill weed, Mrs. Dash, and parsley.

3. Preheat oven to 425. Generously coat fish with mayo and then crumb mixture. Spray a 9×13-inch baking dish with nonstick spray, and place fish in dish. Sprinkle with lemon juice.

4. Bake 10 minutes per inch thick.

5. Serve with lemon wedges.

Three-Bean Salad

YIELD 6 ½-CUP SERVINGS

A ½ cup serving would count as 1 ounce meat, because beans are relatively high in protein.

1 (15 oz.) can red kidney beans, drained	1 small onion, finely chopped
1 (15 oz.) can reduced salt green beans, drained	1 clove garlic, crushed
	1 tbsp cider vinegar
1 (15 oz.) can chickpeas, drained	1 tbsp olive oil
	½ tsp ground cumin seeds

1. Combine beans and chickpeas in a large bowl, and add remaining ingredients.

2. Mix well and chill.

Chicken Sauté

YIELD 4 3-OZ. SERVINGS

One 3-ounce serving would count as 3 ounces meat.

¼ cup olive oil	1 tsp dry mustard
¼ cup lite soy sauce	2 chicken breasts, boned and halved
1 cup dry sherry	2 tbsps olive oil

1. Combine ¼ cup oil, soy sauce, sherry, and mustard to make marinade.

2. Marinate chicken in the refrigerator for at least 1 hour.

3. Sauté drained chicken over medium to high heat in the 2 tablespoons oil for 8–9 minutes on each side.

Spinach Walnut Salad

YIELD 4 SERVINGS

A 1-cup serving would count as 1 serving from the vegetable group.

8 oz. spinach, thinly shredded	2 tbsps olive oil
2–3 scallions, chopped	1 tbsp lemon juice
2 tbsps chopped walnuts	1 tbsp finely chopped mint

1. In a small bowl, combine spinach, scallions, and walnuts.

2. Combine oil, lemon juice, and mint in a small bowl. Mix well. Pour over spinach, toss, and serve.

Baked Turkey Breast

YIELD 6 4-OZ. SERVINGS

One 4-ounce serving would count as 4 ounces from the meat group.

1 stalk celery, sliced

1 medium carrot, sliced

1 medium onion, sliced

2 lbs turkey breast

1 tsp olive oil

1 cup white wine

1 tsp dried thyme

$1/4$ tsp coarsely ground
  black pepper

1. Preheat oven to 375. Place sliced vegetables in the bottom of the roasting pan.

2. Rub turkey with olive oil and place it on top of vegetables.

3. Pour wine over the top and sprinkle with thyme and pepper. Place the pan on the top shelf of the oven.

4. Roast for 40 minutes. Cover and continue cooking for 30 minutes. Uncover and cook for additional 20 minutes.

Roasted Bell Pepper and Olive Pizza

YIELD 12 SERVINGS

Serving size: one wedge; 104 calories; 15.2 grams carbohydrates; 3.2 grams fat

2 large red bell peppers

2 large yellow bell peppers

½ cup sliced green olives

¼ cup chopped fresh parsley

2 tsps drained capers

2 tsps red wine vinegar

¾ tsp olive oil

⅛ tsp black pepper

2 (1 lb), Italian cheese-flavored pizza crusts (such as Boboli) or focaccias

6 tbsps (1½ oz.) freshly grated Parmesan cheese

1. Preheat oven to 350.

2. Cut bell peppers in half lengthwise and discard seeds and membranes.

3. Place bell pepper halves, skin sides up, on a foil-lined baking sheet, and flatten with hand.

4. Broil 15 minutes or until blackened.

5. Place in a zip-top plastic bag and seal.

6. Let stand 15 minutes.

7. Peel and cut into strips.

8. Combine bell peppers, green olives, parsley, capers, vinegar, olive oil, and black pepper in a bowl.

9. Divide the bell pepper mixture evenly among pizza crusts; sprinkle with cheese.

10. Bake at 350 degrees for 7 minutes or until cheese melts. *Cut each into 12 wedges.*

12 | First Steps to Success

AT this point, you should understand the fundamental concepts of cellulite reduction and the basic principles of the exercise program. You should also know how to follow the Purposeful Nutrition Plan for enhanced fat loss during the eight-week training period. You have all the information necessary to significantly improve your cellulite situation, but you may not know how to take the first step in putting it into practice. Knowledge is important, but action is essential. The program doesn't work unless you implement it—and the sooner you start, the better.

If you have access to a good fitness facility, please follow the recommendations in the next section. If you plan to exercise at home, skip ahead to page 191 for your *getting started* guidelines.

Exercising at a Fitness Facility

step 1 Be sure to have your physician's permission before beginning your exercise program.

step 2 Make an appointment with a certified fitness instructor. This should be a cooperative meeting in which you share the components of the cellulite reduction program and the instructor explains the facility operation, equipment utilization, and training procedures. If you are pleased with the instructor, the facility, the equipment, and the exercise atmosphere, schedule your first training session.

step 3 During your first training session, learn how to properly perform the five leg exercises (Leg Extension, Leg Curl, Hip Adduction, Hip Abduction, and Leg Press), the five corresponding stretches (Quadriceps Stretch, Hamstrings Stretch, Adductors Stretch, Abductors Stretch, and Hip Stretch), and the stationary cycle. Do these exercises each training session the first week.

step 4 Begin your second week with instruction for the two midsection exercises (Low Back Extension and Abdominal Curl) and the two corresponding stretches (Low Back Stretch and Abdominal Stretch). Add these exercises to each training session.

step 5 Begin your third week with instruction for the three upper body exercises (Bench Press, Seated Row, and Overhead Press) and the three corresponding stretches (Chest Stretch, Upper Back Stretch, and Shoulder Stretch). Add these exercises to each training session.

step 6 Continue to train consistently, correctly, and progressively. When you feel ready, receive instruction in treadmill use for a weight-bearing alternative (walking, jogging) to stationary cycling. If you prefer, learn how to use the step machine or elliptical trainer for variety in your endurance exercise.

Note: If you must pay a personal trainer for instruction, you may prefer to learn all the equipment/exercises in one or two sessions.

Exercising at Home

step 1 Be sure to have your physician's permission before beginning your exercise program.

step 2 Carefully read the training procedures and exercise protocol for the free weight workouts and stretching exercises. Follow the exercise instructions precisely when performing the strength and stretching exercises.

step 3 During your first training session, familiarize yourself with the dumbbells and bands. Practice proper performance of the five leg exercises (Dumbbell Squat, Dumbbell Lunge, Dumbbell Step-Up, Band Hip Adduction, and Band Hip Abduction), the five corresponding stretches

(Front Thigh Stretch, Front Hip Stretch, Lower Body Stretch, Groin Stretch, and Outer Hip Stretch), and the stationary cycle. Do these exercises each training session the first week.

step 4 Begin your second week by adding the two midsection exercises (Body Weight Trunk Extension and Body Weight Trunk Curl) and the corresponding stretches (Lower Back Stretch and Abdominal Stretch). Add these exercises each training session.

step 5 Begin your third week by including the three upper body exercises (Dumbbell Bench Press, Dumbbell Bent Row, and Dumbbell Overhead Press) and the three corresponding stretches (Chest Stretch, Upper Back Stretch, and Shoulder Stretch). Add these exercises to each training session.

step 6 Continue to train consistently, correctly, and progressively. At week five, switch to treadmill walking/jogging if possible for a weight-bearing alternative to stationary cycling. You may also substitute a step machine or elliptical trainer if this equipment is available.

key factors The following factors are essential for best results whether you train at a fitness facility or at home. Throughout your training program be sure to do the following:

• 1 set of each strength exercise.

• 10 to 15 repetitions of each exercise set.

- Slow movement speed on each exercise repetition.

- Full movement range on each exercise repetition.

- Enough resistance to fatigue the target muscles within 10 to 15 repetitions.

- Increase the resistance slightly upon completing 15 repetitions.

- Exhale during each lifting action, and inhale during each lowering action.

- Hold each stretch for 20 seconds.

- Divide each endurance exercise session into a warm-up segment (low effort), a training segment (moderate effort), and a cool-down segment (low effort).

- Train in comfortable/cool exercise clothing and well-fitted athletic footwear.

- Drink water before, during, and after each training session.

- Follow the nutritional guidelines for sufficient exercise energy and optimum fat loss.

- Report any unusual feelings of fatigue or discomfort to your physician (and fitness instructor, if applicable).

- Enjoy each exercise session by training safely and sensibly.

The No More Cellulite Program Gets Results!

Testimonials

Marion

The Workout for Cellulite Reduction Program did everything I wanted. For one, it changed my way of eating. It was great. I really needed to change my eating habits. I had more energy and felt better on this eating plan. It didn't feel like I was on a diet. On this plan, I actually ate more! In a nutshell, everything improved. I got a lot of comments from members. Someone said I looked "so good" and a lot of people didn't believe how old I was (73). They thought I looked like someone in her early 60s. Also, the members were so glad to see me working out. I would like to continue training, perhaps lose a couple more pounds, but mostly I'd rather add more muscle and tone up more. Because of working out in this program, I believe it led me to better eating habits, and, surprisingly, I found myself able to drink eight glasses of water. I never thought I could drink that much water. Now I look for it. I take it with me in my car. I really would recommend this program to anyone.

During the eight-week cellulite reduction program, Marion lost 19 pounds of body weight and reduced her percentage of body fat by 7 points.

Clara S.

Boy, do I feel great! Not only do my clothes look better and feel better, I have far more energy than I had before I did this workout program. It is like being on an upward spiral. One area of success feeds (excuse the term) another. When you feel good, you want to get out and exercise. Then you gain muscle and burn calories, which makes you feel still better. This program puts you on the road to healthy living.

Clara lost 7 pounds of fat during her eight-week cellulite reduction exercise program. She reduced her percent body fat by 3 points and her hip measurements by 1½ inches.

Danielle

I thought it was a very good workout. The program was well put together, the diet part as well as the exercises. I liked having a trainer pushing me because I know I wouldn't have done it on my own. Having a trainer coax you into doing one more rep and encouraging you helps with consistency. My mother usually cooks for me, and this program forced me to learn how to prepare meals for myself. I feel more energetic, I feel good about myself, more healthy I guess, for example, instead of going to McDonald's, I go get a salad. Because of the menu plan, it's always in the back of my mind that I should be eating healthier, and that's a good thing! After seeing the results of this study, I've continued to work out daily and also eat properly. As far as my appearance, now I feel like I have a shape to my body.

Danielle lost almost 10 pounds of fat and added 1 pound of muscle. Her percent body fat decreased 4 points, and her hip measurement dropped almost 2 inches.

Barbara F.

I think the program is good. I am a health teacher, so I found the diet to be sound because it included the five food groups. People need to be committed to the food in addition to the exercise to lose the weight.

Barbara dropped almost 5 points in her percentage of body fat. She actually lost 8 pounds of fat, gained 2 pounds of muscle, and reduced her hip measurement by 1 inch.

Betty

I really enjoyed the cellulite reduction program. My instructor was a terrific coach who pushed just hard enough so I would get excellent results and not get discouraged from working too hard. My clothes fit better.

Betty reduced her percent fat by 4 points, lost 5 pounds of fat, and added 3.5 pounds of muscle.

Susan L.

I participated in the South Shore YMCA Cellulite Reduction Program during the spring of 2002. I was extremely pleased with my results through the program. I lost 10.5 pounds and improved my muscle tone and energy level.

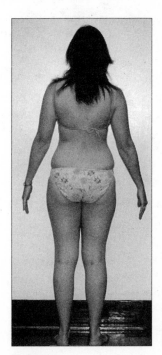 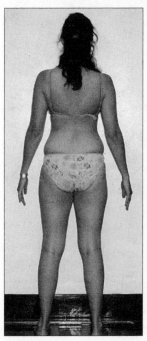

Before   **After**

I was apprehensive about the diet when I first began the program, but I found it to be manageable and effective. I especially enjoyed my workout session with the Y trainer. He was informative, helpful, encouraging, and fun. I learned a lot about strength building and muscle development through our time together.

I have noticed that my clothes fit looser and I feel stronger all over. I have been receiving compliments from friends and colleagues on my appearance. I strongly recommend the program to women who are looking to improve their appearance and need some support to maintain a regular exercise regimen. Knowing that I was meeting with my trainer made it much more difficult to skip a workout session, and with the strong support of Dr. Wayne Westcott and Rita La Rosa Loud, I definitely felt like part of a team.

Susan lost 11 pounds of fat, reduced her percent body fat by 6 points, and decreased her hip measurement by almost 2 inches.

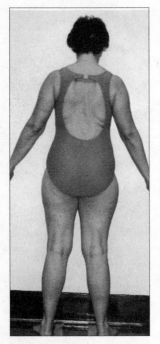 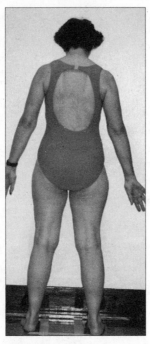

Before   **After**

Marnie

As a participant in the Workout for Cellulite Reduction Program, I must admit that I was skeptical about what results would be achieved. But, the one-on-one training, three days a week, the Nautilus, the cardio, and the diet all helped me arrive at a goal that surprised even me. As I've gotten older, my discipline decreased, while my weight increased . . . this program is the way to go!!! It only took eight short weeks to turn bad habits into healthy commitments.

Marnie lost 10 pounds during her eight-week cellulite reduction exercise program. Her percent body fat decreased by 4 points, and her hip measurements decreased by 2½ inches.

Maria

I think it's a great program. I feel good about it. It's not really a diet; the food you eat is just healthy. It did wonders for me. I learned how to work out and fit my workouts in. I never used to work out before. I never found time. Before I did the program, I was not happy with my appearance at all. I'm very happy to know that because of this program, I lost 13 pounds on the scale, and 14 pounds of fat, plus gained 1 pound of muscle. This program improved my cellulite situation. I do not have as many "pockets" or "holes" anymore.

Maria lost 13 pounds during her eight-week cellulite reduction exercise program. Her percent body fat decreased by 7 points, and her hip measurement decreased by almost 2 3/4 inches.

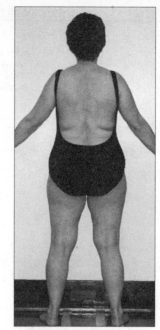 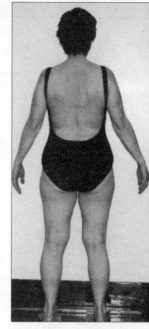

Before   After

Kathleen

It was amazing how much energy I had as a result of the eight-week process. It boosted my self-confidence. I became more knowledgeable and understood the importance of finding and maintaining a balance between a proper diet and an exercise routine. My daily focus and motivational level increased dramatically in my personal and professional life. As a dancer, my flexibility, strength, and

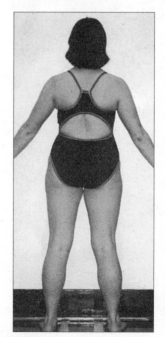 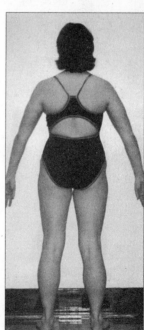

Before   After

energy level improved a lot. I was able to perform at a higher level with much more stamina.

Kathleen lost 6 pounds during her eight-week cellulite reduction exercise program. Her percent body fat decreased by 3 points, and her hip measurement decreased by 2¼ inches.

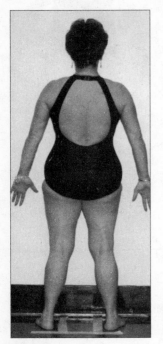

Before

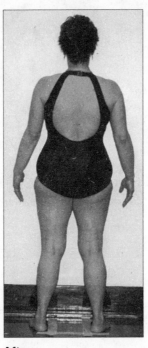

After

Nancy S.

Having tried so many different diets, creams, those type of things, I had the best results with this program. I can now look in a mirror and see the differences in my body, and I like what I see! One of the positive things about the program is that it's only three times per week for one hour and can easily fit into my hectic lifestyle. The diet was very simple to follow. It offers a wide variety of food that never left me hungry. This program has taught me exercise and eating the right food is a way of life.

Nancy lost 9 pounds during her eight-week cellulite reduction exercise program. Her percent body fat decreased by 5 points and her hip measurement decreased by 1½ inches.

Mary

I loved the study. It affected me by helping me lose weight and completely changing my body composition as well as my outlook in life and the way I approach working out. Nothing I've ever tried before has had that much positive effect on my body. I didn't just lose weight, I actually added muscle. Normally I would lose weight and gain it back, lose weight and gain it back. This time I lost it and kept it off because of the added muscle.

Mary lost 7 pounds of fat and replaced 3 pounds of muscle during her eight-week cellulite reduction exercise program. Her percent body fat decreased by 4 points, and her hip measurement decreased 1½ inches.

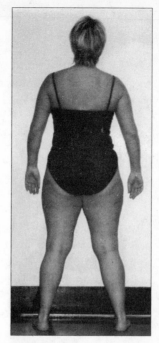 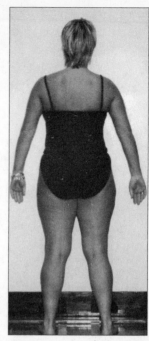

Before   After

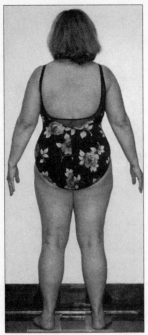

Before

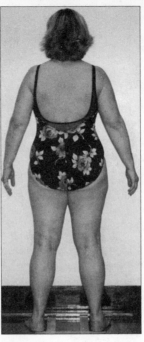

After

Barbara M.

I have participated in this program twice. I wanted to join a program I could commit to; this program was a commitment of three times per week. The exercises were realistic and time-efficient, making it an enjoyable experience. The diet was easy to follow. It's well balanced and offers a variety of foods. I never felt deprived as I have on other diets. My body shape changed very quickly. My clothes fit better almost immediately. My posture is even better. I stand taller now. Also, my thighs are smoother, that's for sure, and that happened the first session, almost immediately! There were times I could see little lumps and bumps through my clothes. Now they've disappeared! I plan to continue to follow this program. I tell everyone, it's a way of life!

Barbara lost 16 pounds of fat and replaced 3 pounds of muscle during her eight-week cellulite reduction exercise program. Her percent body fat decreased by 6 points, and her hip measurement decreased by 2 ³⁄₄ inches.

Tara

The Workout for Cellulite Reduction program offered a structured program that enabled me to reach the goal that I wanted, which was to become more health-conscious. Over the course of the program, I found myself having more energy, being more clear-headed, and motivated to continue exercising.

Tara lost 12 pounds during her eight-week cellulite reduction exercise program. Her percent body fat decreased by 6 points, and her hip measurement decreased by 2½ inches.

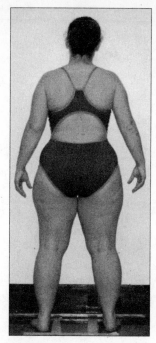
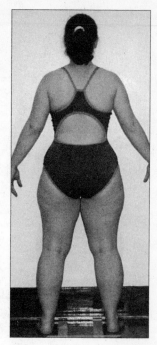

Before   **After**

Basic Stretching Exercises

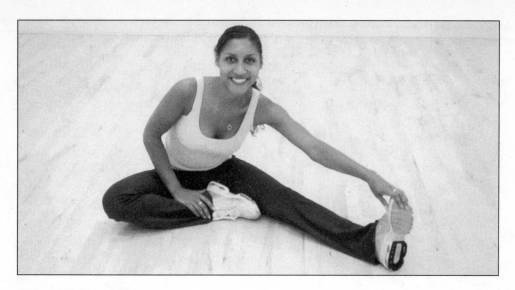

Figure "4" Stretch

Figure "4" Stretch

This stretch resembles the number four and primarily stretches the hamstrings in the rear thigh. Sit on the floor with your left leg straight and right knee bent so your foot touches the inside of your left thigh. Slowly bend at the waist and reach toward your left foot with your left arm. Gently grasp your foot, ankle, or lower leg until you feel a mild stretch in the back of your thigh. Hold this stretch for 20 seconds, then repeat the figure "4" stretch with the opposite leg.

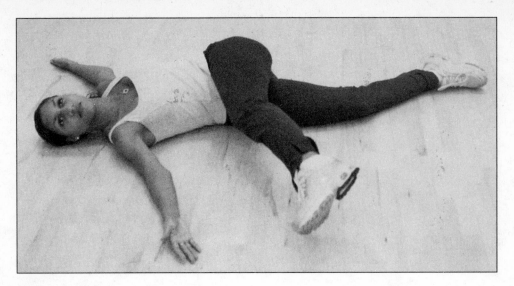

Letter "T" Stretch

Letter "T" Stretch

This stretch resembles the letter "T" and stretches the low back and hip muscles. Lie down on the floor facing the ceiling. Place both arms straight and out by your sides. Lift your left leg directly up and over your body, then lower it toward your right hand. Hold this stretch for 20 seconds. Slowly return your left leg to its original spot and repeat the letter "T" stretch with the opposite leg.

Index

Page numbers in *italic* indicate figures; those in **bold** indicate tables.